Wendkouni Abdoul Fatahou Ouedraogo

Prevalence of swine cysticercosis and risk factors

Wendkouni Abdoul Fatahou Ouedraogo

Prevalence of swine cysticercosis and risk factors

Taenia solium taeniasis in pork consumers in the city of Ouagadougou

Imprint

Any brand names and product names mentioned in this book are subject to trademark, brand or patent protection and are trademarks or registered trademarks of their respective holders. The use of brand names, product names, common names, trade names, product descriptions etc. even without a particular marking in this work is in no way to be construed to mean that such names may be regarded as unrestricted in respect of trademark and brand protection legislation and could thus be used by anyone.

Cover image: www.ingimage.com

This book is a translation from the original published under ISBN 978-620-6-72006-5.

Publisher:
Sciencia Scripts
is a trademark of
Dodo Books Indian Ocean Ltd. and OmniScriptum S.R.L publishing group

120 High Road, East Finchley, London, N2 9ED, United Kingdom
Str. Armeneasca 28/1, office 1, Chisinau MD-2012, Republic of Moldova, Europe
Printed at: see last page
ISBN: 978-620-8-02664-6

DEDICACES

Signing sessions

I am sincerely grateful to all the people who have supported me throughout my university career and who have pulled me up to reach my goal. It is with love, respect and gratitude that :

I dedicate this thesis

A Allah

In the infinite mercy and light of your guidance, I humbly dedicate this work. Your innumerable blessings have been my source of inspiration and strength throughout this intellectual journey. You have awakened in me the strength to understand, explore and deepen the mysteries of your universe. I implore your blessing and grace for all my life.

To the best parents in the world,

This thesis is the fruit of my academic journey, but it is also a reflection of the unconditional love, support and sacrifices you have given me throughout my life. Thank you, Mom, for being there every step of the way. Since elementary school, you've been my teacher, my guide, and you've spared no effort to awaken and develop me. Dad, I also thank you for all these sacrifices.

To my wonderful brothers and sisters, Abdoul Razack, Saad Abdalla and Tasnim Aida

I couldn't have wished for anything better. Without you, I wouldn't be so fulfilled. Thank you so much for your support and help, especially with my studies. You are the best brothers.

To my Grandparents

You are and always will be models for me, thank you for the blessings, the graces, the advice and for your availability. You have never stopped showing me love and I will do anything to make you proud.

ACKNOWLEDGEMENTS

Thanks

We would like to express our gratitude and appreciation to all those who have contributed, in one way or another, to the preparation of this thesis.

To our master Dr Adama ZIDA (MCA)

Our master and thesis director. Thank you for your patience and, above all, for the trust, guidance and invaluable support you have given us in the preparation of this document. You have been a master on whom we have always been able to rely throughout this work. Thank you for your comments, your advice, your dedication and your availability despite your workload.

To our master Dr P. Marcel SAWADOGO (MA)

Our teacher and thesis co-director. Thank you for your kindness and constant availability, which have always aroused our admiration. You were always attentive to the concerns of your students. Many thanks for your patience. Please accept our thanks for the great honor you have done us by agreeing to supervise this work.

To the members of the jury

Thank you for agreeing to evaluate this work and for all your comments and criticisms.

To the staff of Abattoir Frigorifique de Kossodo

Thank you for your warm welcome, your support and the ideas you put forward to help the study run smoothly.

To my paternal and maternal aunts/uncles

I am both happy and proud to have you in my life. **Uncle Issiaka, Zackaria, Aziz, Issouf, Adamou, Omar,** you are and will always remain fathers to me. I will always fight to honor you. Thank you for your moral and financial support and encouragement throughout my university years.

Auntie Safi, Rouki, Binta, Sarata, Setou, I can never thank you enough. Thank you for your support in every way.

To my cousins

Anaradia, Latifa, Ahmed, Nassir, Lamine, Faycal, Rafia, Yasmine, Yasser, Issouf, Kassoum, Balde, Mouna, Balkissa, Souley only the LORD and I know the good you have done me. I am sincerely blessed to have you. May GOD bless you and renew your strength.

To Jeannie, one of my most beautiful encounters

You have been a great support to me. Thank you for your selfless and unconditional love. May the LORD grace us with the happiness we all look forward to. Thank you for existing.

To Amadoum DIALLO,

He who knows me better than I know myself; you spared no effort to be with me when I needed company the most. You have always shown me your love, and I am truly grateful. May the LORD bless your studies and all your endeavors. May he give you the wife you deserve.

To my dear elders and fellow faculty members,

Fayçal Habib, Nackou, Serge, Philippe, Fayçal Diallo, Fatahou, Sidi, Mahomed, Axon, Prisca, Yasmina, Oumaima, Christelle, Sané, Stan, Gilonne, Sapateh, Jeannie, Chaida, Ami, Fabrice thank you for everything. Thank you for your support in one way or another during my university career. I pray that you will be watered as you have watered me and beyond your expectations.

To the brothers and sisters the neighborhood has given me,

Fay, Fabi, Stan, Aziz, Oumar, Ibrahim, Mady, Ali, Saydou how can I not thank you for everything you've done for me. I have always felt like family at your side. May you be richly blessed.

To the late Moustapha OUEDRAOGO

Uncle, I'm here today because of you. From where you are, you must be very proud of me. I pray for the salvation of your soul and that God soothes our still bruised hearts.

To my acquaintances

Dr Elisabeth Kaboré, Dr RAMDE, the staff of the Koulouba pharmacy, Mr Ramdé Brouahiman who, in one way or another, have contributed to my development as a student. You have been a channel and a blessing for me. May the LORD always remember you.

To all my supervisors,

Please accept our gratitude for this modest work.

TO OUR HONORABLE MASTERS AND JUDGES

❖ **To our honourable master and jury president:**

Professor Oumar GUIRA

You are

- ✓ **Full Professor of Internal Medicine at the Joseph KI-ZERBO University Health Science Training and Research Unit (UFR/SDS)**
- ✓ **Internist, CHUYO Internal Medicine Department**

Dear Master,

We are very honored to have you as Chairman of the Jury. You are a master respected by all for your rigor in your work and your availability. The immensity of your scientific knowledge has made you an admired master among students.

Please accept our sincere thanks and deep gratitude.

❖ **To our Honorable Master, Judge and Thesis Director,**

Doctor Adama ZIDA (MCA)

You are

- ✓ **Pharmacist-biologist, former hospital intern in Ouagadougou ;**
- ✓ **Associate Professor of Parasitology and Mycology at the Unité de Formation et de Recherche en Sciences de la Santé (UFR/SDS), Joseph KI-ZERBO University;**
- ✓ **Head of the Parasitology-Mycology and Bacterio-virology Department at the Yalgado OUEDRAOGO University Hospital (CHU-YO);**
- ✓ **Technical Referent for Neglected Tropical Diseases ;**
- ✓ **Director of the Centre National de Recherche et de Formation sur le Paludisme ;**
- ✓ **Technical Director, CNFP**

Dear master,

Not only did you agree to guide our steps, but you also invested a great deal of personal effort in the realization of this work, despite your many requests. Your sympathy, your availability, your rigour in your work and above all your love for research have won our admiration and our attachment to you. It was a great pleasure for us to benefit from your practical teaching and, above all, your practical guidance in drawing up this document. Please accept our sincere thanks and deep gratitude.

May the LORD grant you long life and bless you and your family!

To our honorable master and judge

Dr Mamoudou SAVADOGO (MCA)

You are

- ✓ **Infectiologist ;**
- ✓ **Associate Professor of Infectious Diseases at the UFR /SDS of Joseph KI-ZERBO University;**
- ✓ **LMD pedagogical coordinator.**

Dear master,

It's a great honor and privilege for us to have you as a jury member. We have benefited from your theoretical and practical guidance throughout our university career. Your sympathy, your self-sacrifice, your simplicity, your ability to listen and the interest you show in your students have won us great admiration throughout our studies. While we hope that this work has not fallen short of your expectations, allow us, honourable master, to reiterate our deep gratitude for the invaluable teachings we have been fortunate enough to benefit from. Thank you, dear master, for everything.

May God, in His grace, grant you a full life, bless you and fulfill you beyond your expectations.

To our honorable master and thesis co-director,

Doctor Patindoilba Marcel SAWADOGO

You are

- ❖ **Pharmacist, Former Intern at the Hospitals of Burkina Faso ;**
- ❖ **Assistant Professor of Parasitology-Mycology at the UFR/SDS of Joseph Ki-ZERBO University;**
- ❖ **WHO expert in malaria microscopy;**

Dear master,

We are delighted that you have honored us by agreeing to co-supervise this work. Despite your busy schedule, you have unreservedly agreed to accompany us on this thesis. Thank you for your availability and your sound advice on how to improve this work. Thank you from the bottom of our hearts for your attentive ear, your kindness and your patience. Please find in this work the testimony of our gratitude and the assurance of our respectful sentiments.

God bless you, your family and all your endeavours, and grant you a long and happy life!

WARNING

"By deliberation, the UFR/SDS has decided
that the opinions expressed in the dissertations
to be presented must be considered as the
authors' own and that it does not intend to give
them any approval or improbation".

TABLE OF CONTENTS

TABLE OF CONTENTS

INTRODUCTION AND PROBLEM STATEMENT

INTRODUCTION AND PROBLEM STATEMENT

Taeniasis is an intestinal infection caused by adult tapeworms of the *Taenia* genus, including *Taenia solium*, *Taenia saginata* and *Taenia asiatica*. While humans are the only definitive host for each of these species, *Taenia solium* is of particular importance in terms of public health.[21]

Taenia solium is a zoonotic parasite affecting mainly pigs, and occasionally other animals. In humans, the adult tapeworm develops in the small intestine, causing taeniasis.[100]. Neurocysticercosis, a severe form of human infection in the larval stage, can cause neurological disorders, including seizures, with potentially fatal consequences. Swine cysticercosis, although often asymptomatic in pigs, causes significant economic losses through carcass seizure and depreciation in animal value[94].

Prevention of human cysticercosis involves the detection and treatment of human tapeworm carriers, public health education, appropriate sanitary facilities, adequate personal hygiene and good food hygiene. Collaboration between veterinary and human health authorities is essential to prevent and control *T. solium* transmission. In Burkina Faso, the prevalence of *T. solium* taeniasis and the risk factors associated with pork consumption are major public health issues.

Unfortunately, in the city of Ouagadougou, there is a lack of precise data on the prevalence of *T. solium* taeniasis and the risk factors for human contamination associated with pork consumption. For this reason, this study aims to determine the prevalence of porcine cysticercosis in the AFO and to identify risk behaviours for human contamination associated with pork consumption. The results of this study will be essential in guiding prevention and control measures for this parasitic infection, thereby helping to improve public health.

PART ONE: GENERAL INFORMATION

I. GENERAL INFORMATION ON TENIASIS

I.1. Background

In antiquity, Hippocrates (460-380 B.C.) already distinguished three types of human parasitic worms: tapeworms, roundworms and<<ascarids>>.The first category corresponds to cestodes (tapeworms), which Hippocrates described as very long, expelled in rings and with egg-filled segments. In his *Historia animalium*, Aristotle (384-322 B.C.), who can be considered the founder of parasitology, is the first to describe pig ladreria or cysticercosis, particularly in the tongue. This description was taken up by Oribasius (325-403) and Albert the Great in his *De animalibus* (1193-1280). A case of cysticercosis was described in an Egyptian mummy who lived during the Ptolemaic period [305-30 BC]. [62].

Rumber first described human cysticercosis in 1558. The Italian Marcello Malpighi (1628-1694), founder of microscopic anatomy, described the tapeworm scolex (1681) and the *Taenia solium* larva, clearly establishing the relationship between the two stages (1687). The English zoologist Edward Tyson (1651-1708) was the first to recognize that the anterior end of tapeworms is found in the slender region of the worm. He also described the scolex and hooks.

Nicolas Andry (1658-1742), a Lyonnais physician and parasitologist, published a treatise on the generation of worms in the human body. He divided human worms into 14 categories according to their location in the body. The true founder of helminthology was the German Karl Asmund Rudolphi (1771-1832). He named the larval stage of *T.solium Cysticercus cellulosae*, because of its distribution in subcutaneous tissue. It wasn't until the 19th century that it was experimentally demonstrated that the pig cysticerci is the larval form of *T.solium* (Kuchenmeister) and the beef cysticerci is the larva of *Taenia saginata* (Leuckart).[59].

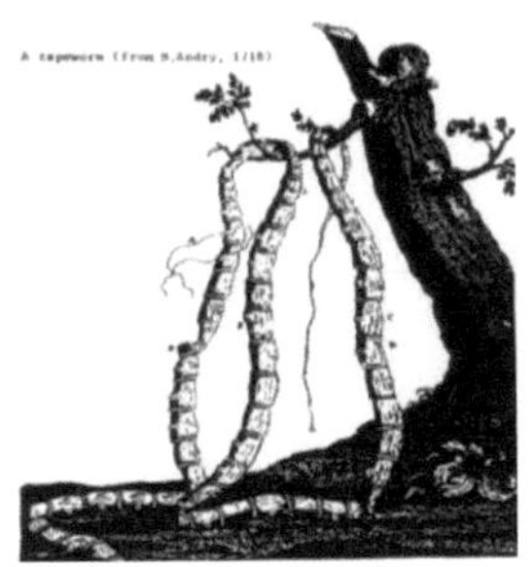

I.2 EPIDEMIOLOGY

I.2.1 Pathogen

Taenia solium is a parasite belonging to the flatworm phylum, more specifically to the Cestoda class. Commonly known as *taenia*, it is found in the human intestine. It can reach measurements of up to 4 meters and is responsible for the development of taeniasis and cysticercosis (rare). [14].

In its life cycle, it has an intermediate host, which is often pork. As a result, consumption of undercooked pork is one of the main sources of infection. Taeniasis is an easily treatable and eradicable disease. However, it can sometimes become chronic and even lead to intestinal obstruction, the consequences of which can be very serious.[67].

In the proglottids of *Taenia solium*, both male and female reproductive organs can be appreciated. It is said to be hermaphroditic. These communicate with each other, so that the process of fertilization and egg formation can take place.

Taenia solium is a heterotrophic organism. This means that it does not have the capacity to synthesize its own nutrients, so it must feed on substances manufactured by other living beings. [25].

When in the human intestine, the parasite feeds on intestinal chyme by osmosis. It absorbs mainly carbohydrates. It's also worth mentioning that through the microvilli that surround its body, they optimize this absorption process.

This parasite, like all parasites, causes an imbalance in the body, leading to disease. *Taenia solium* It is responsible for two diseases: taeniasis, which is caused by the adult parasite, and cysticercosis, which is caused by cysts that form in various body tissues, such as the brain, muscles and lungs[27].

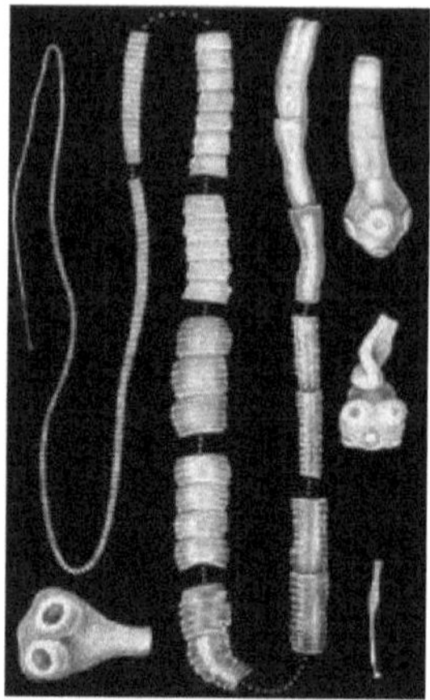

Figure 1 *Taenia solium* specimen.*[35]*

I.2.1.1 Taxonomy

The taxonomic classification of *Taenia solium* is as follows:

- Estate: Eukarya
- Kingdom: Animalia
- Phylum : Platyhelminthes
- Class: Cestoda
- Order: Cyclophyllidea
- Family: Taeniidae
- Genre: *Taenia*
- Species: *Taenia solium*

I.2.1.2 Morphology

Taenia solium specimens vary in color from white to ivory. In terms of length, they are quite long, reaching up to 8 meters. This organism consists of a body and a head or scolex.

The scolex is generally pyriform in shape and features four round structures called suction cups. At the anterior end of the scolex, a protuberance can be seen with a double ring of hooks. This structure is called a rostellum. Between the scolex and the body of the parasite is a space known as the neck.

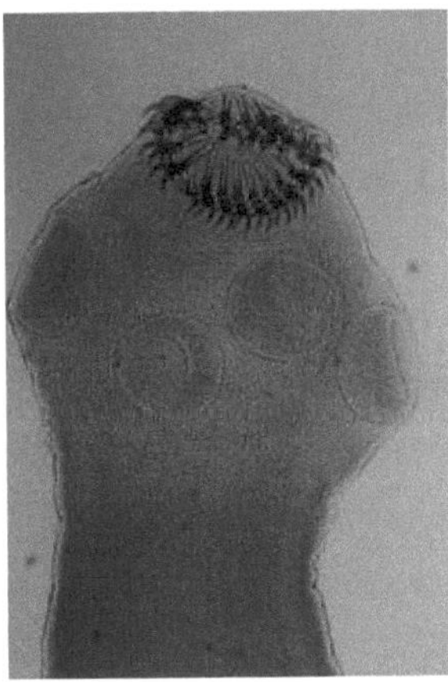

Figure 2 *Taenia solium* scolex: the suction cups and rostellum are visible.*[69]*

Like all plathelminths, *Taenia solium* has a flattened body, which is divided into segments called proglottids. Mature proglottids are quadrangular in shape and also have unilateral genital pores. They feature both male and female reproductive structures.

Proglottids in a more distal position are gravid. Morphologically, length predominates over width. These proglottids have a large uterus with a central branch consisting of several branches. These are full of eggs, numbering between 50,000 and 60,000. The last proglottid ends in a hole called the caudal foramen.

Eggs are spherical in shape, with a diameter of around 31 to 41 microns. Structurally, they have several membranes, including the yolk, present only in immature eggs. The yolk covers the embryophore. Similarly, the oncosferal membrane covers the Hexacanto embryo.

The hexacanth embryo is simply the larval stage of the cestodes. In this, the presence of three pairs of hooks is visible.[54]

I.2.1.3. Bio-ecology (reproductive habitat and pathogenicity)

I.2.1.3.1. Habitat

Depending on the stage of their life cycle, porcine tapeworms inhabit a variety of environments. Pre-adult and adult tapeworms can be found in the small intestine of mammals.

Egg-bearing segments of proglottids are found in the host's feces and in the external environment where feces are excreted.

Unfortunately, not enough research has been carried out on the subject of embryos in the outdoor environment. Consequently, it is difficult to determine which habitat embryos prefer. However, embryo survival is known to be affected by temperature.

If the environment is colder than 10 degrees Celsius or warmer than room temperature (37 degrees Celsius), it's easy for eggs to succumb.

The next stage of tapeworm development is the oncosphere, which occurs in the intermediate host pig.

The oncosphere's habitat is the intestines and tissues of the pig host, and its cysticercal stage persists in the pig's muscles and brain. The cysticercal form can also survive in a human host, residing in muscle and brain [93].

I.2.1.3.2. Nutrition

Taenia solium is a tapeworm parasite that lives in the small intestine of humans as the definitive host, and of pigs as an intermediate host. As an adult, *Taenia solium* absorbs nutrients by attaching to the wall of the host's small intestine and absorbing digested food through its body surface.

In the larval stage, *Taenia solium* forms a cyst (bladder worm) in the tissues of the pig. The bladder worm absorbs nutrients from the host's tissues by diffusion through its body surface.

When a human eats undercooked pork containing cysts, the cysts are digested and the larvae are released into the human small intestine. The larvae then attach to the wall of the small intestine and develop into adult tapeworms.[81]

I.2.1.3.3. Reproduction

Taenia solium has both sexes. The reproductive organs of both sexes resemble those of the liver fluke. Each proglottid after the first 200 has a set of reproductive organs. The male reproductive organs develop first in each proglottid, followed by the advent of the female organs.

- **Male reproductive organs**

Numerous spherical testes are scattered along the length and width of the proglottis. Each testicle contains a small efferent duct. Efferent ducts from adjacent regions combine to form larger ducts. These larger ducts connect to the vas deferens or main testicular duct.

The vas deferens is contoured, transverse and extends to the left or right lateral edge of the proglottitis. The apex of the vas deferens is narrow and enters a narrow protuberant process, the cirrus or penis, before opening into a cup-shaped genital atrium via the male gonopore.

The base of the cirrus is enclosed in a muscular capsule called the cirrus sac.

- **Female reproductive organs**

In the posterior region of the proglottis, there are two pairs of bilobed ovaries or germaria. The two lobes are of unequal size and are located on either side of the midline. The oviducts are composed of numerous branched tubules that originate from the ovaries. The two oviducts converge to produce a median oviduct.

At the posterior edge of the proglottid, a single yolk gland or yolk gland composed of a few lobules opens into the median oviduct via the yolk duct. Numerous spherical shell glands (also known as Mehlis glands) are located around the yolk duct, and the shell gland ducts drain into the oviduct on the side of the yolk duct.

The ootype refers to the specialized part of the oviduct where the shell gland ducts and yolk ducts are accessible. The ootype penetrates anteriorly into a median, elongated, blind uterus. A fertilizing or spermatic duct emerges from the ootype. The anterior part of the spermatic duct forms the seminal receptacle. The vagina emerges from the receptaculum seminalis, moves forward and laterally, and opens into the atrium. In mature or pregnant proglottids, the uterus enlarges, branches out and fills with fertilized eggs. As a result, other structures are diminished and altered.

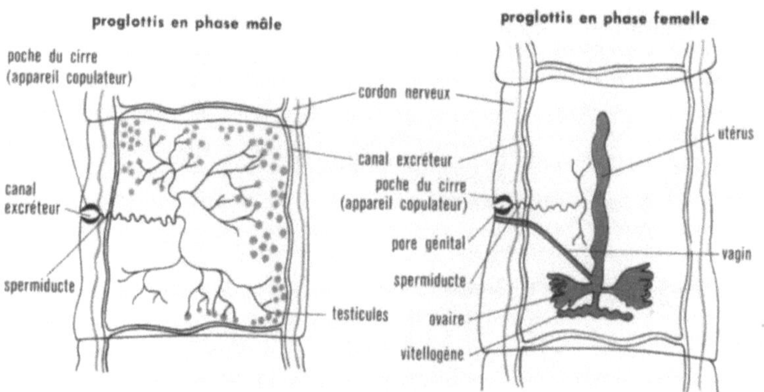

Figure 3 Male and female reproductive systems of *Taenia solium*[2]

I.2.1.3.4. Pathogenicity

Adult worms and cysts are pathogenic. Adult worms are less pathogenic. Their armed scolex may cause slight irritation or inflammation of the intestinal mucosa. Cysts (Cysticercus cellulosae) are more pathogenic. They cause a serious disease cysticercosis in humans, mainly cysts can be found in the skin, skeletal muscles, eyes and CNS.[39]

- **Disease in pigs**

In most cases, the disease is asymptomatic. At the very start of infestation, pigs present mild diarrhea due to irritation of the intestinal mucosa. Once the cysticerci have settled in, signs of myositis may be observed, resulting in locomotion or mastication problems. Encephalitis and even epileptic seizures have been described when cysticerci localize in the brain. Death can occur suddenly in the event of massive infestation of the heart.[49]

- **The disease in humans**

Intestinal taeniasis

Most of the time, the infection is asymptomatic. In symptomatic cases, clinical symptoms are non-specific and mild, and include nausea, abdominal discomfort, hunger pains, weight loss, chronic indigestion, etc.

Less frequently, vomiting, headache and diarrhea are present in a few cases. [5].

Cysticercosis

Cysticercosis is infection by the larval stage of the parasite. Humans contract the infection through fecal oral contamination with *T. solium* eggs from tapeworm carriers, or through self-infection.

Clinical manifestation depends on the organ affected; neurocysticercosis and ophthalmic cysticercosis are associated with significant morbidity [76].

Extra neural cysticercosis

Subcutaneous cysticercosis appears as small, painless, mobile nodules commonly found on the arms or chest. After a few months, or even years, the nodules become swollen, tender and inflamed, then gradually disappear. Muscle cysticercosis is a causal finding, appearing as dot-shaped or ellipsoidal calcifications. In rare cases, very massive parasitic loads enlarge the patient's limbs (muscular pseudohypertrophy).The heart is another occasional location, infected in around 5% of cases.The patient's cardiac cysticercosis is asymptomatic [95].

Ophthalmic cysticercosis

This condition occurs in 20% of cases. Most cysts are found in the vitreous, subretinal space and conjunctiva. The condition can present as iritis, ureitis and palpebral conjunctivitis. Cysts in subconjunctival or subretinal sites may present as slow-growing nodules mistaken for tumors. Occasionally, subretinal ocular cysts can lead to blindness due to retinal detachment[8].

Neurocysticercosis

The parasite generally infects the CNS, causing neurocysticercosis as a clinical disorder. After entering the CNS. Cysticerci cause symptoms due to a mass effect or by blocking the circulation of cerebrospinal fluid, most symptoms are the direct result of the inflammatory process that accompanies cyst degeneration. Symptoms and signs are varied and non-specific. Seizures are the most frequent presentation, and usually represent the main or only manifestation of the disease. Seizures occur in 50-80% of cases of parenchymal brain cysts or calcifications. The disease also manifests as intracranial hypertension, hydrocephalus or both in 20-30% of cases. The syndrome is linked to the localization of parasites in cerebral ventricles or basal cisterns blocking CSF circulation, and is caused by several different mechanisms: the presence of the parasite itself, ependymal inflammation or residual fibrosis. Occasionally, a cyst becomes larger than usual, acting in the same way as a tumoral mass (giant cyst).

These giant cysts compress adjacent brain structures, causing localized deficits and intracranial hypertension. Motor deficits may also occur due to edema secondary to cystic degeneration, or following stroke complicating the infection.

In children and adolescents, acute encephalic presentation may occur, more likely in females than in males. Massive non-encephalic forms also occur. Spinal compromise occurs in 1% of adult cases, presenting with a compressive manifestation.[24]

I.2.2. Final host

Man is the definitive host of *Taenia solium*, which means that adult worms live and reproduce inside human intestines[25,80]

I.2.3. Intermediate host

Taenia solium's intermediate host is the pig and occasionally man (human cysticercosis).[86].

Experimental studies following a strict protocol have shown that cats and dogs can be temporary hosts for *T. solium*, although the worm does not develop into the adult stage. A gibbon was experimentally infected and a gravid proglottid was recovered, demonstrating that it can act as a definitive host. Pigs are the native intermediate hosts, while humans and dogs can also act as intermediate hosts for the parasite[83].

I.2.4. Mode of contamination

Humans become infected through ingestion of raw or undercooked meat contaminated with *T. solium* cysticerci. [27]He accidentally harbors the cysticerci:

- Either after ingesting eggs with vegetables or contaminated water;
- Or by faecal peril through contact with a carrier and ingestion of eggs;
- Or by self-infestation from oncospheres produced by the tapeworm host itself. Self-infestation leads to continuation of the cycle in the same host. This can occur through fecal soiling (dirty hands), as well as through digestion of rings brought up by their own movements and intestinal antiperistalsis. The latter eventuality is formidable, as it releases a large number of embryos and leads to generalized cysticercosis. In this case, the initial contamination of man is due to the absorption of pork, and teniasis precedes cysticercosis.[92].

I.2.5. Output path

Adult *Taenia solium* can leave the human small intestine in two different ways:

- Anus: Adult *Taenia solium* consists of several segments called proglottids. These segments, containing mature eggs, break off and are expelled from the body with the stool. The segments resemble small grains of rice and may be visible in the stool or on the patient's underwear.[17]

- Mouth: it has been reported, albeit rarely, that tapeworm solium segments can emerge from the human mouth during vomiting or regurgitation. This is an extremely rare situation, but it can happen.[74]

I.2.6. Evolutionary cycle

The cycle is heteroexenic, with man as definitive host and pigs as intermediate host. In the case of tapeworm, the mode of contamination is uncooked pork. In the case of human cysticercosis, infection may occur through self-infestation or by ingesting food contaminated with eggs.[54]

Pigs become infected by ingesting foodstuffs contaminated with human faeces, containing embryophores of *Taenia solium*. The embryo is released in the pig's digestive tract, under the effect of gastric juice, and crosses the intestinal mucosa with its hooks. By blood or lymphatic circulation, it arrives at the organs of predilection, which are the eye, the brain, striated muscles, but also the heart and the tongue, where it transforms into a larva.[72]

The Cysticercus *cellulosae* larva (translucent vesicle containing an invaginated scolex with four suckers and a rostrum) encysts.

In humans, by ingesting contaminated pork, the larva evaginates in the jejunum, attaches to the digestive mucosa and develops into an adult within 2 to 4 months. The detached mature proglottids are immobile and evacuated into the external environment when they pass stool. Once in the external environment, the rings are lysed, releasing the embryonated eggs.

Ingestion of food contaminated with human faeces containing *Taenia solium* embryophores, or the upwelling of gravid proglottids in the stomach, which release eggs (self-infestation), leads to the development of human cysticercosis.

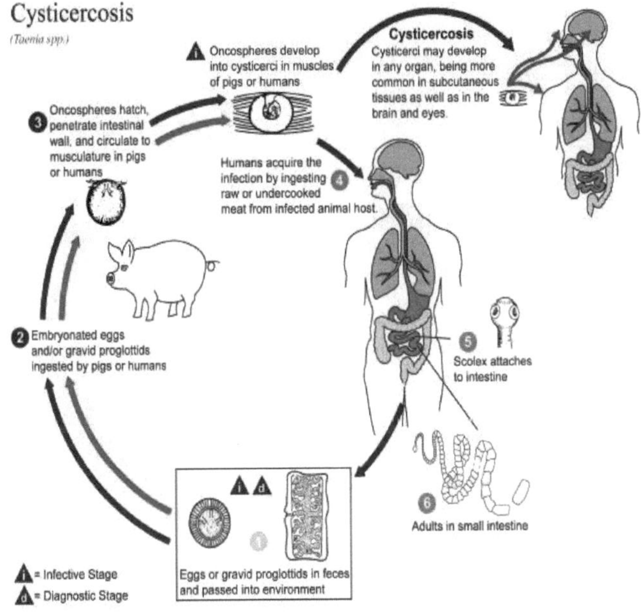

Figure 4_T.solium_ evolutionary cycle[1]

I.2.7. Favoring factors

✓ Consumption of undercooked or raw pork: The main route of infection for _Taenia solium_ is ingestion of the larvae present in contaminated pork. If the meat is undercooked, the larvae can survive and infect humans.

✓ Lack of hygiene: Failure to observe hygienic measures, such as inadequate hand washing after contact with contaminated faeces, can increase the risk of accidental ingestion of _Taenia solium_ eggs.

✓ Poor sanitary conditions: Unfavorable sanitary conditions, including limited access to drinking water and adequate sanitary facilities, can favor the spread of parasitic infections, including _Taenia solium_ tapeworm.

✓ Lack of awareness and education: Lack of knowledge about the risks associated with eating undercooked pork and about appropriate preventive measures can contribute to the transmission of _Taenia solium_ taeniasis.

✓ Pork rearing and slaughtering practices: Pork rearing and slaughtering practices that do not comply with appropriate hygiene standards can lead to contamination of meat by *Taenia solium* larvae.[19].

I.2.8. Epidemiological parameters and geographical distribution

T. solium is a cosmopolitan parasite whose transmission is linked to poor hygiene conditions, common in developing countries. Its frequency is still poorly estimated. *T. solium* is found with high prevalence rates in Latin America, Asia, Black Africa and the Indian Ocean. According to the WHO, 2.5 to 5 million people are carriers of the adult worm and 50 million of cysticercal larvae; cysticercosis is thought to be responsible for 50,000 deaths per year.[67] By harboring the adult worm in their intestine, humans play a major role in the dissemination of the parasite in the environment. Carriers of *T. solium* become infected through ingestion of raw or undercooked pork, which retains viable cysticerci. *T. solium* transmission also requires that pigs have access to human faeces. These conditions (lack of faecal hygiene, precarious pig-rearing conditions with wandering pigs and consumption of undercooked pork) are frequently found in rural areas of endemic countries. Conversely, these conditions are no longer found in most industrialized countries (Europe, North America and Australia), and cysticercosis is practically non-existent in Muslim countries.

❖ Industrialized countries :

The majority of cases reported in developed countries are due to immigration from endemic countries [12,18]. In Europe, *T. solium* is rare [30]. Indeed, a recent review covering the period 1990-2011 provides the following information [101]. Of 846 cases of cysticercosis reported in the literature, 522 were autochthonous (including 70.1% from Portugal) and 324 imported (including 17.6% from travellers and 74.7% from migrants). The majority of imported cases came from Latin America. They were diagnosed in Spain (47.5%), France (16.7%) and Italy (8.3%). The Iberian peninsula remains an endemic zone, especially in northern Portugal and western Spain. Imported cases are rare in Canada and Australia, but are now frequent in the United States as a result of large-scale immigration from Latin America. The first alert concerning this re-emergence of *T. solium* in the USA came in the 1990s, when several cases were described in an Orthodox Jewish community in New York, with an estimated seroprevalence rate of 1.3% - a surprisingly high figure for a community whose religion forbids the consumption of pork. [51]. Their employees, recent immigrants from Latin America, were subsequently identified as the source of the infection [82]. Subsequently, 221 deaths were attributed to cysticercosis during the period 1990-2002[88]. Overall, among the non-endemic countries traditionally considered, it was in the USA that the increasing prevalence of neurocysticercosis was first identified. During the 1980s and 1990s, there was a massive immigration of people from Latin America, as well as an increase in the number of neurocysticercosis patients, especially in the southern states from Texas to California, along the Mexican border. Neurocysticercosis then appeared in other states. Finally, autochthonous cases began to be described, now accounting for around 5% of neurocysticercosis patients in the USA. Over 5,000 cases have been reported in the USA in recent years.

❖ In Latin America

Cysticercosis is a long-standing problem in Latin America [64]. Numerous human prevalence studies have been carried out: Colombia (1.8-2.2%), Brazil (3.0-5.6%), Mexico (1.3-10%), Peru (7.1-26.9%), Honduras (15.6-17%), Ecuador (2.6-14.3%), Guatemala (10-17%), Bolivia (22%) and Venezuela (4-36.5%). Average seroprevalence is consistently high, at around 10%. The prevalence of neurocysticercosis varies from 1% to 22% (average rate: 7%), based on CT and MRI findings. The prevalence of porcine cysticercosis is extremely variable: from less than 2% to over 75%. Guatemala, Honduras, Mexico and Peru show the highest rates[24,64]. The prevalence of the disease varies from 0 to 33.3%, and transmission still appears to be active in rural areas of Mexico [53]. The contamination of house floors by Taenia eggs has also been studied; the highest values were recorded on kitchen floors and in springtime[34]. Fecal contamination still represents a risk in rural communities.

❖ In Africa and Madagascar

An almost complete ignorance of the *T. solium* cycle involving pigs (cysticercosis) and men (taeniasis and cysticercosis) has been systematically reported in studies conducted in Africa[9,41]. *T. solium* is probably widespread in most African countries where pigs are raised in the wild and pork meat is consumed. However, there are many countries where no information is available. Although epilepsy is a major problem in African countries, often associated with neurocysticercosis, ultimately few studies have been undertaken on the tapeworm/cysticercosis complex [73].

Cysticercosis has been described in West and Central Africa (Cote d'Ivoire, Togo, Mali, Benin, Nigeria, Cameroon, Central African Republic, etc.). In Cameroon, the first cases of human cysticercosis were described in the Western Province in 1985[99]. Cameroon is one of the Central African countries where the tapeworm/cysticercosis complex has been extensively studied in humans and pigs. In the western province of Cameroon, human cysticercosis has been estimated at between 0.7% and 2.4%. A study of epileptic patients revealed a high prevalence rate of 44.6%.[99]. The prevalence of porcine cysticercosis, measured by tongue sampling, is 6.1%; it ranges from 11.0 to 21.8% by ELISA tests [70]. In East and Southern Africa, the teniosis/cysticercosis complex is an emerging problem, mainly linked to increased pig production in Kenya, Uganda, Zambia and Zimbabwe[47,66]. The rate of swine cysticercosis has been estimated at around 10%. Other studies report that neurocysticercosis and epilepsy are public health problems in Burundi and the Democratic Republic of Congo[102].

In Madagascar, the first cases were described at the beginning of the twentieth century[75]. Seroprevalence of active cysticercosis has been estimated at between 7 and 21%: values are below 10% in coastal regions (Mahajanga and Toamasina) and higher in central regions (Antananarivo, Fianarantsao), where pig farming is more important [77,100]. In a seroepidemiological survey carried out in the port of Mahajanga, the prevalence of cysticercosis was estimated at 19%. [49]. Cysticercosis has been identified as a risk factor for epilepsy[4].

In Asia, the prevalence of *T. solium* is difficult to estimate due to the simultaneous presence of *T. saginata* and *T. asiatica*. Nevertheless, *T. solium* is present in the most populous countries, such as Indonesia, China, India and Vietnam[71,96]. *T. solium* infection is less common in the Philippines, Thailand, Malaysia, Bangladesh and South Korea. The disease is rare in the Arabian Peninsula, Afghanistan, Iraq, Iran and Pakistan [64]. In China, the policy of opening up the market, implemented nationwide in 1989, led to a sharp increase in the number of small butchers and private slaughterhouses, where there is no rigorous meat inspection. Since then, more and more cases of taeniasis and cysticercosis have been recorded in provincial hospitals. Five provinces are hyper-endemic for porcine cysticercosis: Sichuan, Yunnan, Guizhou, Qinghai and Inner Mongolia. Yunnan is particularly hard hit, with prevalence rates ranging from 0.5 to 2.8% and human teniosis rates from 13.2 to 34.7[10]. In Henan, following a six-year control program, *T. solium* teniosis fell by 90.8% and cysticercosis by 96.8 [98]However, infection in pigs, and consequently pig-to-human transmission, is resistant to this type of campaign. Veterinary control is the first step in limiting transmission. Vaccination of pigs is another possibility[13,44]. Several organizations are currently working on the implementation of control programs: the Peru Cysticercosis Working Group[32]the Cysticercosis Working Group in Eastern and Southern Africa [40]the Network for

taeniasis/cysticercosis and echinococcosis in Asia and the Pacific Region[35] and more recently the Cysticercosis Working Group in Europe[97]. These programs must support joint action between doctors, veterinarians and biologists. They require the political support of affected countries, as well as that of international bodies such as the WHO and FAO.[20]. Above all, they must combine several actions: mass treatment, veterinary control, vaccination campaigns and education.[23]

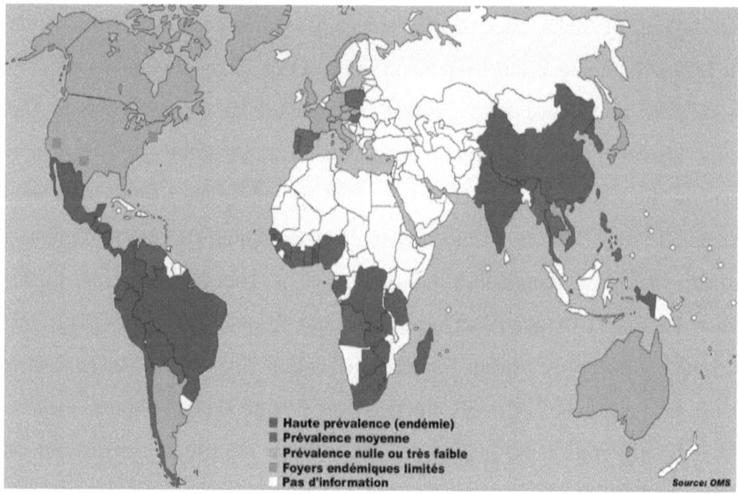

Figure 5 Geographical distribution of *T.solium* (source WHO 2015)

I.3 Biological diagnosis

I.3.1. Circumstances of diagnosis

The circumstances in which *Taenia solium* taeniasis is diagnosed may vary according to the patient's symptoms and epidemiological circumstances. Here are a few situations that could lead to a diagnosis of *Taenia solium* taeniasis:

- **Presence of worm segments in the** stool

Segments of *Taenia solium*, called proglottids, may be visible in the patient's stool. These segments resemble small pieces of flat white ribbon and can be spotted with the naked eye.[29]

- **Self-diagnosis**

In some cases, patients may notice worm segments in their stool or around their anus. They may suspect a parasitic infection and consult a healthcare professional for diagnosis and appropriate treatment.[29]

- **Gastrointestinal symptoms**

People infected with *Taenia solium* may experience gastrointestinal symptoms such as abdominal pain, nausea, vomiting, diarrhea or loss of appetite. These symptoms may lead to medical examinations to establish an accurate diagnosis.[10]

- Neurological **symptoms**

If *Taenia solium* larvae migrate into the central nervous system, they can cause neurological symptoms such as headaches, convulsions, visual disturbances, behavioral changes or signs of meningitis. In these cases, medical imaging tests, such as computed tomography (CT) or magnetic resonance imaging (MRI), can be performed to identify larval brain damage.[12]

- **Exposure to** endemic **areas**

If the patient has traveled to or lives in an area where *Taenia solium* infection is endemic, the diagnosis of taeniasis may be considered depending on the prevalence of infection in that region.[7]

I.3.2. Non-specific biological modification

It is based on HES of variable magnitude, generally peaking between the 5th and 10th week after infestation, with a return to normal within 3 to 5 years. In cerebral localization, CSF examination shows elevated blood eosinophilia, hyperalbuminorachia and hypoglycorachia. Serology does not always give good results. Parasitological examination of stools reveals *T. solium* rings and embryophores.[6]

I.3.3. Parasitological diagnosis

Coprological methods

They involve the detection of eggs and/or ovigerous proglottids in faeces. In general, the sensitivity of fecal examination is not very high. Several diagnostic techniques combined (flotation, sedimentation) can detect 91 to 97% of infestations, while a single technique can detect 50 to 78% of cases. During passage through the anal sphincter, eggs are released and deposited around the peri-anal surface, where they can be collected directly (scotch tape technique) for direct microscopic examination. Proglottids are expelled intermittently with the faeces of carriers. A single microscopic examination is therefore sometimes insufficient. Patients should be asked if they are aware of harboring the adult worm.

I.3.4. Immunological diagnosis

Immunological diagnosis of *Taenia solium*, also known as swine tapeworm, can be made using various serological tests. Here are some of the tests commonly used to diagnose *Taenia solium* infection:

Anti-T. *solium* antibody assay: This test measures the presence of specific antibodies to *Taenia solium* in the patient's blood. It can be performed using techniques such as ELISA (enzyme-linked immunosorbent assay) or immunoblot.

Immunoblot: This technique uses proteins extracted from *Taenia solium* to specifically detect antibodies to this organism. It is often used to confirm a positive ELISA result. Indirect immunofluorescence test (IFI): This test is based on the detection of specific antibodies to *Taenia solium* in patient serum. Antigens from *Taenia solium* are attached to a solid support and react with antibodies present in the sample. When antibodies are present, specific fluorescence is observed.

Western blot test: This test is similar to the immunoblot and is often used to confirm the positive results of other serological tests. It detects specific antibodies to *Taenia solium* proteins.

It should be noted that these immunological tests detect the presence of antibodies produced by the immune system in response to infection by *Taenia solium*. However, they cannot differentiate between an active infection and a previous infection or exposure to the organism. Consequently, additional tests, such as medical imaging (CT scan, MRI) or stool analysis for *Taenia solium* eggs, may be required to confirm the diagnosis. It is advisable to consult a healthcare professional for an accurate and appropriate diagnosis.[6]

I.3.5. Molecular diagnosis

Molecular diagnosis of *Taenia solium,* also known as swine tapeworm, is generally performed using molecular biology techniques. Here are some of the methods commonly used to diagnose this parasitic infection:

PCR (Polymerase Chain Reaction): PCR is a technique used to specifically amplify *Taenia solium* DNA fragments present in a sample. Parasite-specific primers are generally used to detect and amplify the parasite's DNA. This method is highly sensitive and can detect small quantities of *Taenia solium* DNA. PCR (real-time quantitative PCR): PCR is a variant of PCR that quantifies parasite DNA in the sample. It uses specific primers and a fluorescent marker to measure the quantity of amplified DNA in real time. This method is also highly sensitive, enabling precise detection and quantification of *Taenia solium* DNA.[36]

LAMP (Loop-mediated Isothermal Amplification): LAMP is a DNA amplification method that takes place at a constant temperature. It is fast and sensitive, and requires no sophisticated equipment. LAMP uses specific primers to amplify *Taenia solium* DNA and can be used in the field for rapid diagnosis.[36]

DNA sequencing: DNA sequencing can be used to specifically identify *Taenia solium* from amplified DNA. This technique makes it possible to determine the parasite's genetic sequence and confirm its identification.[11]

I.3.6. Histological diagnosis

Histological diagnosis of *Taenia solium* involves examining tissue samples taken from the patient to detect the presence of specific features of the organism. The main methods used for the histological diagnosis of *Taenia solium :*

Biopsy: A biopsy is the removal of a sample of tissue suspected of being infected by *Taenia solium.* In the case of *Taenia solium* infection, the most common sites for biopsy may be muscle, the central nervous system or ocular tissue. The tissue is then fixed, cut into thin sections and stained before being examined under the microscope. Specific staining: Various staining techniques can be used to highlight the specific characteristics of *Taenia solium* in tissue samples. For example, hematoxylin-eosin (HE) staining can reveal the presence of larvae, cysts or other characteristic lesions associated with *Taenia solium* infection.

Microscopic observation: Stained tissue samples are observed under the microscope by a pathologist to identify the characteristic structures of *Taenia solium*. These structures may include worm segments, hooks, scolex, proglottids (tapeworm segments) or cysts containing *Taenia solium* larvae. Histological examination confirms the presence of *Taenia solium* in the patient's tissues, and can provide information on the extent of infection and damage to surrounding tissues. However, it is important to note that histological examination alone is not sufficient for a complete diagnosis. Other complementary tests, such as serological tests, stool analysis or medical imaging examinations, may be required to confirm the diagnosis of *Taenia solium* infection. [6]

I.4. Therapeutic principle

I.4.1. Purpose of treatment

Remove adult worms and eggs from the intestine.

I.4.2. Resources

The reference treatment is Praziquantel (Biltricide®), a single-dose anti-helminth (effective against worms). It works by blocking glucose metabolism.

Niclosamide (Trédémine ®), also a single dose. However, a few precautions are necessary: it should be taken after a light meal and followed by a laxative 2 h later.[28]

I.4.3 Indications and dosage

❖ **Praziquantel**

Therapeutic indications

It now represents the reference for *T. solium.*

Its main indications are parasitic infections caused by trematodes, including :

- o Bilharziasis: *Schistosoma haematobium, Schistosoma intercalatum, Schistosoma japonicum, Schistosoma mansoni,*
- o Distomatoses*: Clonorchis sinensis, Opisthorchis viverrini, Paragonimus westermani*

The usual dosage is 10 mg/kg in a single dose for *T. solium* taeniasis, but has shown a 100% success rate on *T. solium* at a dose of 2.5 mg/kg[65]. Side effects are rare: headache, asthenia, arthralgia, abdominal pain.

❖ **Niclosamide**

Treatment of *T. saginata, T. solium, Diphyllobotrium latum* and *Hymenolepis nana* tapeworms.

Dosage: prescribed at a dose of 2 g for adults, and at a dose reduced by half or a quarter for children, this product requires a special method of administration:

- ✓ Fasting from the previous day,
- ✓ Take two tablets, chew for a long time and then swallow with very little water,
- ✓ Wait one hour on an empty stomach,
- ✓ Take two more tablets, chew for a long time and then swallow with very little water,
- ✓ Wait another three hours before eating.
- ✓ **NB**: Surgery may be recommended for the treatment of complications. Kalkan et *al.* 2013 successfully removed tapeworms endoscopically from

the stomach. Other endoscopic approaches that have been used include injecting drugs into the wall of the small intestine, allowing tapeworms to detach from the intestinal wall and be excreted in the stool.

I.4.4. Post-therapy biological monitoring

Post-treatment biological monitoring is primarily aimed at assessing treatment efficacy and detecting early reinfection. Laboratory tests commonly used for biological monitoring of taeniasis include microscopic examination of stools to detect the presence of parasite proglottids in the stool. A negative stool examination after treatment suggests that the treatment has been effective. It is recommended to carry out a stool examination in the weeks following treatment. If the examination is negative, a further examination should be carried out several weeks later to confirm the absence of reinfection.

Serological tests can be used to detect antibodies produced in response to infection. These tests can be useful for confirming past infection, but are not sensitive for detecting early reinfection.[28]

I.5. Prevention

Given the significant economic and public health impact of this parasite, it is essential to find effective means of prevention. Prophylaxis is based on interrupting the epidemiological cycle in the definitive host (man) and the intermediate host (pig).

I.5.1. Purpose

Breaking the chain of transmission

I.5.2. Strategy

I.5.2.1. Individual strategy

Individual prevention involves first and foremost health education, with regular hand hygiene to combat faecal peril in humans, particularly after contact with animal carcasses, followed by the consumption of well-cooked meat (infectious forms are rapidly killed at temperatures of over 60°C), or else frozen beforehand at 10°C for 10 days, or for a few days at -20°C to -25°C. Salting can be an effective way of sanitizing meats (although a 20° Baumé brine is required). Ionizing radiation treatments (20,000 to 60,000 rads or cobalt 60) can also be used, but are rarely used as flatworm larvae seem less sensitive to this sterilization technique. The use of human excreta as fertilizer in agriculture should also be avoided.[16]

I.5.2.2. Collective strategy

The general preventive measures to be adopted are :

- Raising awareness of the importance of food hygiene and proper cooking practices

- Fighting illegal slaughter

- Combating animal straying

- Construction of latrines (to prevent egg dispersal)

- Deworming animals

- Improving sanitation and hygiene

- Promote sewage systems or build latrines to prevent eggs from being dispersed.

- Do not use untreated human faeces to fertilize meadows and pastures

- Treatment of infected subjects.[7]

- Avoid eating pork

PART TWO: OUR STUDY

OBJECTIVES

I. OBJECTIVES

I.1 General objective

To determine the prevalence of porcine cysticercosis at the Ouagadougou cold-storage abattoir, and the risk behaviors for taeniasis among pork consumers in the city of Ouagadougou.

I.2. Specific objectives

1. To determine the prevalence of porcine cysticercosis at the Ouagadougou refrigerated abattoir.
2. Describe the socio-demographic characteristics of pork consumers in Ouagadougou
3. To assess the general knowledge of Ouagadougou pork consumers about *T. solium* tapeworm.
4. Describe the eating habits of pork consumers in the city of Ouagadougou
5. Identify the various risk factors for taeniasis

MATERIALS AND METHODS

II. MATERIALS AND METHODS

II.1 Study framework

Our study took place in the Centre region (specifically in the city of Ouagadougou) one of Burkina-Faso's 13 administrative regions. It has an estimated population of 3,032,668 according to the 2019 general population and housing census (RGPH), with a density of 1,081 inhabitants/Km^2 and covers an area of 2,085 Km^2 . It is made up of a heterogeneous population both ethnically and geographically. The Centre region is subdivided into 7 departments: Komki-Ipala, Komsilga, Koubri, Ouagadougou, Pabré, Saaba and Tanghin-Dassouri. Ouagadougou is the administrative capital and largest city in Burkina-Faso.

In terms of health, the region boasts five (5) Health Districts (DS), four (4) University Hospitals (CHU), two (2) Medical Centers with Surgical Antenna (CMA) and one hundred and sixty-two (162) Health and Social Promotion Centers (CSPS), according to data from the Direction régionale de la santé center.

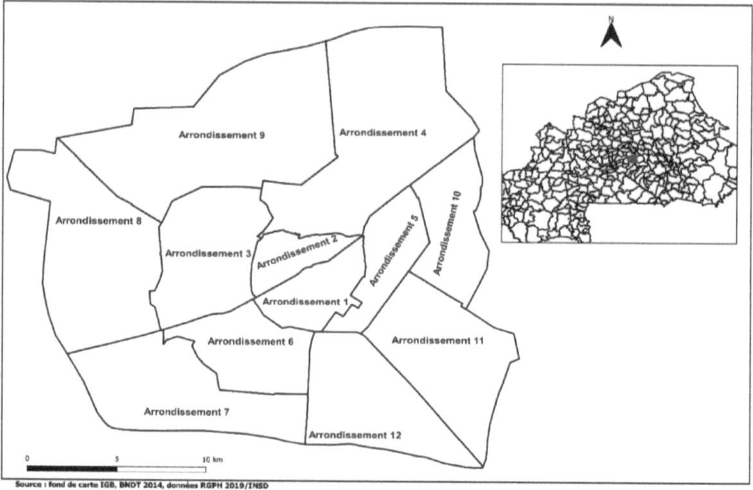

Figure 6:Map of the Ouagadougou commune (central region)

The first part consisted of a parasitological study carried out at the Abattoir Frigorifique de Ouagadougou (AFO), the largest meat production site in Burkina-Faso.

AFO is a public industrial and commercial establishment (EPIC). It has legal and civil personality, and financial autonomy. Commissioned on August 7, 1975, its production capacity was 13,000 tons of meat per year. Following an expansion in 1981, this capacity was increased to 15,000 tonnes per year. In 1987, it was transformed into a Mixed Economy Company (S.E.M) with capital of 10 million CFA francs. The slaughterhouse was built in response to Burkina Faso's need to rationally exploit its livestock by marketing meat. Since its creation, the plant has been a service provider, operating as a municipal abattoir.

The Ouagadougou abattoir covers an area of 74 ha and is located in the Kossodo industrial zone on the Kaya road, 7 kilometers from downtown Ouagadougou.

In terms of infrastructure, the slaughterhouse is made up as follows:

- A central building (the largest) housing the offices, slaughter lines, cold rooms and machine room.
- A building housing the workers' washrooms, stores, canteen and emergency treatment room.
- A small sanitary slaughterhouse for the emergency slaughter of sick or suspect animals. It is equipped with an incinerator for the destruction of dangerous meat.
- A rendering plant to process blood, bones and unhealthy meats into meal.
- A garage, a livestock market for the sale of live animals, a shed for breaking heads, a pit equipped with a filter for decanting wastewater.
- Last but not least, a solar water heater used to scald pigs and clean slaughter rooms.

Management of the AFO has been entrusted to SOGEAO (AFO's management company).

The second part of the study was a survey of beef consumers in the city of Ouagadougou.

II.2 Study period

The study took place over sixteen months, from January 2022 to April 2023.

II.3 Type of study

This was a descriptive cross-sectional study carried out in Ouagadougou at the AFO and among pork consumers.

II.4. Study population

The slaughterhouse survey included all pig carcasses slaughtered and inspected by veterinary officers. All carcasses relevant to the study period were taken into account.

The population survey concerned pork-eating residents of Ouagadougou, who are likely to be exposed to the risk of taeniasis if they eat contaminated meat.

II.4.1. Inclusion criteria

All pigs slaughtered during the study period and pork consumers aged 15 and over, living in the city of Ouagadougou and having consumed pork at least once in the three months prior to the survey, were included in the study.

II.4.2. Exclusion criteria

We excluded from the study all people who were unable to understand the questionnaire or who had incompletely completed it. Also excluded were people who responded to the online questionnaire but did not live in Ouagadougou.

II.5 Sampling and sample size

II.5.1. Sampling

As the sampling frame of pork consumers (complete list) is not available, probabilistic methods cannot be used, but rather empirical methods. In our case, we used the standard unit method. This method involved defining precise criteria, namely pork consumption and being at least 15 years old, and then stopping the collection once the sample size had been reached.

II.5.2. Sample size

According to the Schwarz method, the standard equation for calculating sample size is as follows:

$$Taille\ de\ l'échantillon = \frac{z^2 p * (100\% - p)}{e^2}$$

- Z=Statistic of the normal distribution centered reduced for n greater than or equal to 30. It is 1.96 for a confidence level of 95%,

- P= Pork consumers in the city of Ouagadougou

- 1-p=proportion of individuals not involved in the study (non-consumers of pork)

- e=Margin of error = 5%.

As p is not known from existing statistics, we will use 50% as the percentage of pork consumers in the city of Ouagadougou. Applying this formula gives a minimum size of 384 pork consumers. To account for partial or total non-responses, the final sample size was 404 consumers.

II.6. Equipment

- Pigs
- Humans

❖ **Tools**

We used a survey form addressed to pork consumers in Ouagadougou. To assess the prevalence of cysticercosis at Ouagadougou's refrigerated abattoir, we used the following materials:

- A pair of boots

- A white coat
- A knife
- A flashlight
- Disposable latex gloves
- A smartphone for taking photos.
- Scorecards

II.7. Data collection

Data collection took place at the Ouagadougou cold-storage abattoir, and the information gathered was the results of post-mortem examinations. These mainly concerned the presence or absence of cysts and their location.

Data collection then took place in the form of a survey to gather targeted information, structured according to a predefined questionnaire tailored to the research objectives; the questionnaire was administered online; collection sheets were also drawn up for mobile collection. The information collected concerned the socio-demographic characteristics of the respondents, their knowledge of taeniasis, and their culinary habits.

II.8. Description of the study

II.8.1. Parasitological study

The parasitological study was carried out at the AFO over the period January 2022 to January 2023, and involved all pigs slaughtered during this period. We joined the animal health unit in charge of post-mortem inspection of carcasses and the various organs of predilection for cysticerci.

II.8.1.1. General principles of post-mortem inspection

Post-mortem inspection was carried out as soon as the carcass had been dressed, as certain lesions could disappear or develop over time. Apart from the skin, no part of the animal was removed from the premises until the post-mortem inspection had been carried out. It is vital to maintain the link between a carcass and its offal until inspection is complete, so an effective labelling system was needed for both carcasses and offal. Carcasses deemed fit for human consumption were clearly marked immediately after inspection. The mark must be clearly visible and self-explanatory;

When the abnormality was localized, a partial rejection of the carcass or an organ was performed, and only the affected part and tissues in the immediate vicinity were rejected and classified as unfit. In the case of generalized infection, the entire carcass was seized.

II.8.1.2. The various stages of post-mortem inspection

The specificity of meat inspection was 38.7%. All professional and technical skills were used to apply observation, incision and palpation techniques.

- Carcass preparation: the skin and internal organs, such as the liver, were removed to enable inspectors to visualize the muscles and deep tissues of the carcass.
- Visual inspection: inspectors carried out a thorough visual inspection of the muscles, using a flashlight to identify potentially infectious cysts.
- Palpation: inspectors also used palpation to detect cysts not visible to the naked eye. They gently squeezed the muscles to detect any areas of different consistency or small mass formations.
- Marking and classification: the carcass and viscera of an infested animal had to be differentiated according to their level of infestation. Generalized infection means that two or three cysts are found in each cut of the masticatory muscles, heart, diaphragm and its pillars, and that two or three cysts are found in the muscles visible during dressing operations. In the event of moderate or light infestation, corresponding to a small number of dead or degenerated cysticerci, the carcass is kept for a maximum of 10 days at -10°C.

All positive and negative results during our study period were recorded in our collection sheets.

II.8.1.3. Characteristics of the cysticerci

On post-mortem inspection, the cysticerci appeared as :

- Small white lesions in the muscles (cysticerci two to three weeks after infection).
- Clear, transparent vesicles, 5 mm x 10 mm (infectious cysticerci, 12 to 15 weeks after infection);
- Opaque, pearl-like cysts (after 15 weeks of infection);
- Degeneration, caseation and calcification of cysts (after 12 months or more of infection).

II.8.2. Survey

The online questionnaire initially attracted 250 responses. We then drew up a paper questionnaire in order to reach all segments of the population. This questionnaire was also administered at random in the markets and neighborhoods of Ouagadougou to people meeting the survey criteria, resulting in a further 154 responses.

II.9. Variables collected

The following variables were collected during the study:

Socio-demographic variables: age in years, gender, occupation, level of education and place of residence.

Clinical variables: History of *T. solium* taeniasis, history of abdominal or neurological symptoms following pork consumption.

Eating habits: average cost of meat consumed per week, meat cooking methods, place of purchase, consumption of smoked or grilled roadside meat, consumption of imported meat, consumption of raw or undercooked meat.

II.10. Ethical and administrative considerations

Before starting the study, we submitted the research protocol to the ethics committee, which approved it. We obtained written approval from the Direction

Régionale de la Santé du Centre and the Abattoir Frigorifique de Ouagadougou, after explaining the objectives and methods used.

Informed consent was sought from participants prior to their inclusion in the study. Data were collected anonymously under conditions guaranteeing confidentiality.

The results will be disseminated by appropriate means, in particular in the structures included and scientific journals.

II.11. Data analysis plan

II.11.1. Data quality control

Data was collected and stored on survey cards. At the end of each day, we systematically checked all completed forms to ensure that they had been filled in correctly, and corrected any errors on the same day.

II.11.2. Statistical analysis

All data collected was entered, processed and analyzed using Epi Info 7.2 and Microsoft Excel 2019. Calculations of positional parameters such as averages, standard deviations and the creation of tables were carried out using Epi Info software, while the tables and graphs were formatted using Excel.

RESULTS

III. RESULTS

III.1 Parasitological study in the intermediate host

III.1.1. Overall prevalence of porcine cysticercosis

During the study period, a total of 4923 pigs were slaughtered. There were multiple supply zones. The most important are the North, North-Central and East, which are relatively large production centers.

Pouytenga, Kaya, Djibo and Fada contributed to the AFO.

The pigs were of local breeds and produced in two systems: extensive (around 87%) and intensive (around 13%).

We had a total of 67 cases of cysticercosis, giving an overall prevalence of 1.4%. Prevalences of (2.7%) and (2.0%) were recorded in March 2022 and April and December 2022 respectively. In January and February 2022 we recorded a prevalence of (0.6%). This is shown in figure 7.

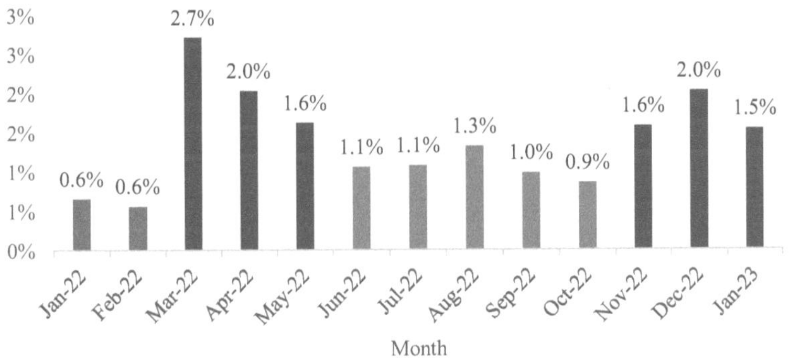

Figure 7 Prevalence of swine cysticercosis by month

III.1.2. Frequency of swine cysticercosis by month

Frequencies of 13.4% were observed in March 2022 and December 2022; a frequency of 13.4% was observed in January 2022 and February 2022 (3.0% of cases).

The table below shows these results.

Table I Monthly incidence of porcine cysticercosis at AFO

Periods	Total number of controlled slaughters	Number of cases	Frequency
Jan-22	308	2	3,0%
Feb-22	360	2	3,0%
March-22	332	9	13,4%
Apr-22	345	7	10,4%
May-22	370	6	9,0%
June-22	378	4	6,0%
Jul-22	556	6	9,0%
August-22	378	5	7,5%
Sept-22	406	4	6,0%
Oct-22	468	4	6,0%
Nov-22	317	5	7,5%
Dec-22	445	9	13,4%
Jan-23	260	4	6,0%
Total	**4923**	**67**	**100%**

III.1.3. Distribution of cysticerci according to organs

On post-mortem inspection, cysticerci were sought in the various organs, namely the carcass, liver, heart and tongue. These analyses showed that the heart was the most infected organ, with a total of 55 cases out of 67. Few cysticerci were found in carcasses (5 cases) and tongue (2 cases). It should also be noted that no cysticerci were found in the lungs. These elective locations can be broken down as follows.

Table II Distribution of cysticercosis cases by location

Cysticercosis (localization)	Workforce	Frequency
Carcass	5	7,46%
Liver	1	1,49%
Heart	55	82,09%
Language	2	2,99%
Other	4	5,97%

Total	67	100%

III.2. Sociodemographic survey for men

III.2.1. socio-demographic characteristics

❖ The sex

The total number of study participants was 404. Fifty-seven point four percent (221/404) were female. The sex ratio (M/F) was 0.82.

❖ Age

The average age of the study population was 33 ±12 years. The youngest was 15 and the oldest was over 66. 43.1% (174/404) of the pork consumers surveyed were aged between 26 and 35, while 6.7% (27/404) were over 65. This is shown in the table and figure below.

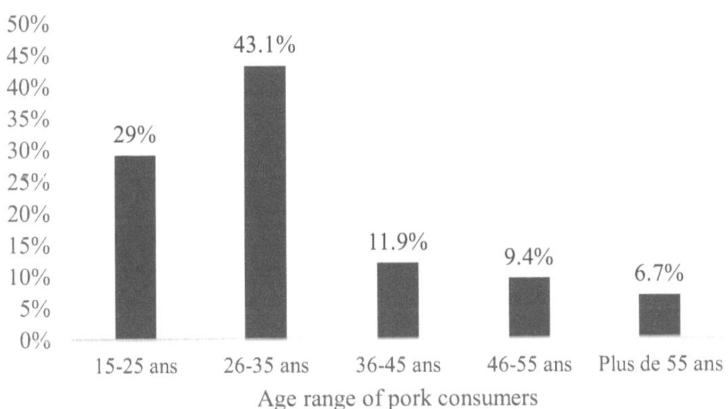

Figure 8 Age distribution of study population

❖ Study level

Respondents were heterogeneously distributed according to education level. The proportion of the population with higher education was 68.8% (278/404). For the other population groups, i.e. secondary, primary and non-educated, the figures were 11.4% (46/404), 7.7% (31/404) and 12.1% (49/404) respectively. The figure below shows the results.

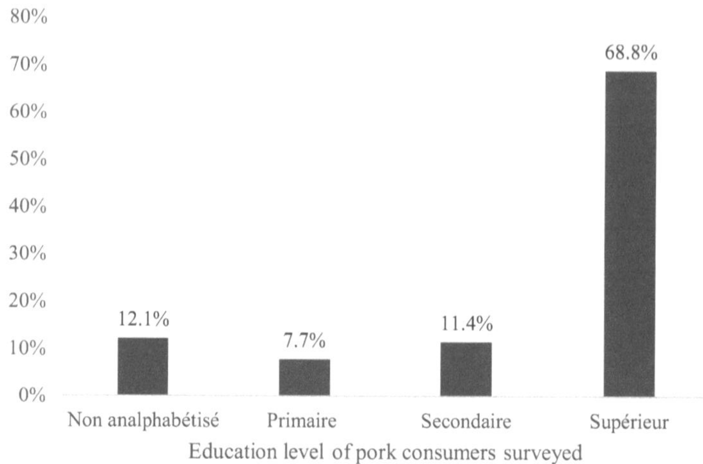

Figure 9 Distribution of study population by level of education

❖ Profession

The distribution of the study population according to profession was also diverse. In our study sample, housewives were the most numerous with 32.2% (130/404), followed by pupils and students with 31.4% (127/404) and civil servants with 12.9% (52/404). The results are presented in the table below.

table III Distribution of study population by profession

Profession	Workforce	Frequency
Artisan	12	3,0%
Retailer	52	12,9%
Pupil/Student	127	31,4%
Civil servant	52	12,9%
Housekeeper	130	32,2%

Liberal profession	6	1,5%
Retirement	6	1,5%
Private-sector employee	17	4,2%
Unemployed	2	0,5%
Grand total	**404**	**100%**

III.2.2. General knowledge of the study population

It was found that 84.2% (340/404) of respondents had knowledge of the risk of eating raw or undercooked meat, and of the existence of zoonoses transmitted to humans by pork. This gender breakdown comprises 84.7% (103/183) of the total number of men and 83.7% (184/221) of the total number of women surveyed. This is summarized in the graph below.

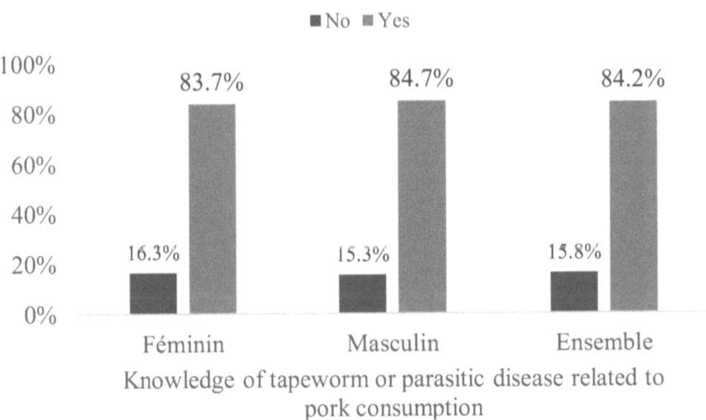

Figure 10 Knowledge of parasitic diseases associated with pork consumption

Our study also enabled us to assess the population's knowledge of *T. solium* taeniasis in humans. In general, we noted an acceptable level of knowledge, but the risk of contamination remains in view of certain practices identified in the study population, which may be a source of contamination and dissemination of the disease throughout the population.

Of those surveyed, 84.2% (340/404) said they were aware of the risks associated with eating undercooked or raw pork, and 15.8% (64/404) of the study population had no knowledge of the routes of transmission of taeniasis.

The majority of study participants (55%, 222/404) were unaware of the causative agent (*T. solium*) of human tapeworm and porcine cysticercosis. We also obtained a high proportion of the study population, i.e. 63.9% (258/404), who were unaware of the symptoms of tapeworm in humans.

44.6% (180/404) had no knowledge of how to prevent tapeworm infection.

III.2.3. Clinical history

Of the consumers surveyed, 65.8% (266/404) reported having experienced one or more clinical signs after eating pork. These symptoms were essentially digestive disorders such as abdominal pain, diarrhea, constipation, nausea and vomiting, and some neurological signs such as convulsions and headaches attributed to the ingestion of poorly cooked food, particularly pork. The frequency of these gastrointestinal disorders is summarized in the figure below.

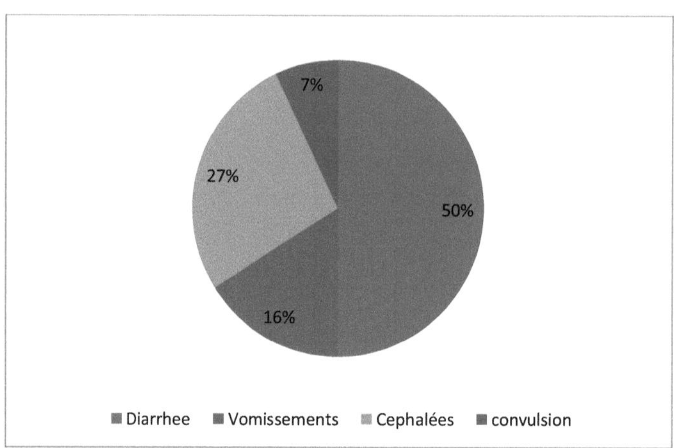

Figure 11:Frequency of disorders

History of *Taenia solium* taeniasis

It was shown that a sizeable percentage of participants had previously been diagnosed with Teniasis. This represented 9.7% of the study population, i.e. 39 of the 404 people surveyed.

III.2.4. Eating habits

❖ Pork consumption frequency

Assessing the frequency of pork consumption enabled us to group consumers into three categories. Of our study population, 10.1% or 41/404 consumed pork frequently (more than ten times a month), 67.6% or 273/404 consumed pork occasionally (at least five times a month) and 22.3% or 90/404 consumed beef rarely (less than once a month, generally during ceremonies). These results are presented in the table below.

Table IV Frequency of pork consumption

Frequency of pork consumption	Workforce	Frequency
Occasionally	273	67,6%
Rarely	90	22,3%
Frequently	41	10,1%
Grand total	404	100%

❖ Place of meat purchase

Meat purchase locations varied. The majority of the study population (213/404) purchased meat from delicatessens, 22.0% (89/404) had no fixed place of purchase and 9.4% (38/404) purchased from local butchers. This is summarized in the table below.

Table V Place of purchase of pork meat

Where to buy pork	Workforce	Frequency
In charcuterie	213	52,7%
Wherever we can find it	89	22,0%
At the local butcher's	38	9,4%
Itinerant butchers	36	8,9%
Breeders	28	6,9%
Grand total	404	100%

❖ **Meat inspection requirements**

Of the 404 respondents, only 29% (117/404) required meat to be inspected by qualified veterinary services before purchase, compared with 71% (287/404) who had no meat inspection requirements.

❖ **Meat cooking techniques**

The people who took part in the study used several domestic techniques for preparing meat. These included boiling, baking, grilling and barbecuing. These results are presented in the table below.

Table VI Meat cooking techniques

Pork cooking technique	Workforce	Frequency
In the oven	301	29,45%
Cooking in oil	299	29,26%
Water cooking	184	18,00%
Barbecue	120	11,74%

Frying	116	11,35%
Steam	1	0,10%
Smoke	1	0,10%
Grand total	1022	100%

❖ **Consumption of imported meat.**

Out of a total of 404 people, 79% (319/404) consumed imported meat (sausage, ham, pâté) and did not usually reheat it before consumption.

❖ **Consumption of undercooked or raw meat**

In the study population, 48.5% (196/404) said they had eaten undercooked or raw meat. The figure below illustrates this result

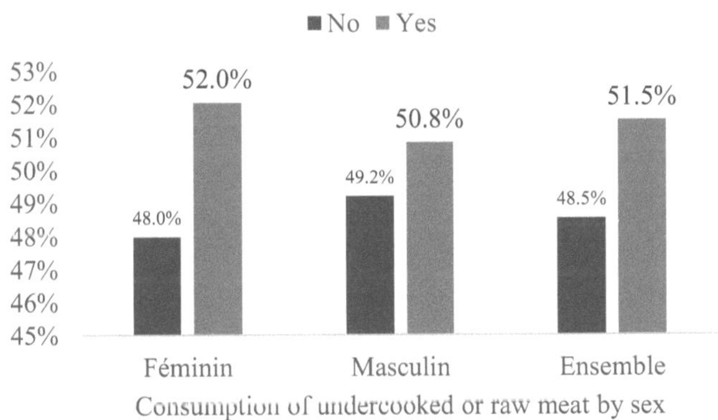

Figure 12 Consumption of undercooked or raw meat by gender

DISCUSSION

IV. Discussion

Our study was conducted in the city of Ouagadougou from January 2022 to January 2023. Following a review of the literature on *T. solium* taeniasis, we became aware of the various dangers and the impact on public health and the economy that this neglected disease could cause, particularly in developing countries with poor sanitation, extensive pig production systems, lack of routine meat inspection practices and high rates of clandestine slaughter. A generally benign pathology that often goes unnoticed, tapeworm disease can have a number of life-threatening complications. Human cysticercosis is a public health problem, responsible for 30% of epilepsy cases.[99]. The lack of data at national level has prompted in-depth studies on the subject, as well as the need to set up national surveillance and control programs for tapeworm and cysticercosis. All these elements were the basis for our choice of subject.

Our objectives were to determine the overall prevalence of porcine cysticercosis at the Ouagadougou cold-storage abattoir, to describe the socio-demographic characteristics of the study population, to assess the population's general knowledge of *T. solium* taeniasis, and finally to describe their different eating habits in order to identify the various risk factors for taeniasis. The categories of consumers, their food preferences for forms of cooked pork meat, the activity and frequency of this consumption were thus better characterized.

IV.1. Study limitations and difficulties

The first difficulty in our study was the night-time slaughter times. We had to go to the slaughterhouse every evening to attend the various inspections, which was complicated by the different courses we had to take during the day. We were helped in this by the entire inspection team, so as not to lose any data.

We were also unable to determine the prevalence of porcine cysticercosis according to animal age, sex and exact origin. This was partly due to the large number of animals slaughtered per day, which made it difficult to take pre- and post-slaughter data, and partly to the nocturnal slaughter times.

Another limitation of this study was the technique used to test for cysticerci, which generally has low sensitivity. According to a number of publications, this technique can only diagnose 30% of cases. [91]of actual cases of cysticercosis. For example, 15.6% detection sensitivity was reported by Eichenberger et *al.* in 2013[104]. In another study, a very low detection sensitivity (0.54%) for meat inspection was reported, whereas the actual prevalence was estimated at 42.5% in Belgium in 2018[105]. This low sensitivity could be linked to the limited number of incisions that can be made due to marketing issues associated with gross mutilation of carcasses and a high probability of contamination (Wanzala et *al.*, 2013)[106]. Consequently, the actual prevalence of porcine cysticercosis could be higher than reported here (1.4%), which could further underestimate the economic and public health impacts in the region. Another limitation of the study is the use of respondents' historical recall to assess history of exposure to human taeniasis; some individuals may suffer from information recall bias that could exceed or underestimate the true extent of the problem. This was particularly evident by the fact that some people who did not consume raw meat reported having had tapeworm in the past. A history of infection should be verified with appropriate tests targeting the general human population.

IV.2 Parasitological study

The overall prevalence of porcine cysticercosis in our study using the post-mortem inspection technique of 1.4% was very close to that achieved by MOPOUNDZA et *al.* in the Kinsoundi slaughter area in Brazzaville using the same technique, which reported a prevalence of 1.69% in 2019.[52] These results are similar to those obtained by Ahossi (2012) for the period 2008 to 2010, which are 1.22% and 1.44% respectively for the Communes of Klouékanmé and Dogbo.

Similar prevalences have also been reported in other regions. Another study conducted by Mwabonimana et *al.* in 2020 also revealed a 1.8% prevalence of swine cysticercosis in western Keneya. The authors also observed that prevalence was higher using the Ag-ELISA test (3.8%) on farms and 5.3% on slaughter tables.

In this study, the prevalence of porcine cysticercosis at post-mortem inspection (1.4%) is higher than the prevalence observed at tongue inspection (1.04%) by Ahoussi in 2012. This could be explained by the fact that post-mortem inspection detects both light and heavy infestations, whereas tongue testing more easily detects heavy infestations. This study's prevalence on post-mortem examination (1.4%) is only slightly lower than the 2.2% observed by Gonzalez et *al.*[31] in 2004. It is much lower than the prevalences of 5.6% and 4.6% reported respectively by Eshitera et *al.*[21] in 2012 in Kenya and Porphyre et *al.*[68] in 2015 in Madagascar. It is low compared with those reported in Zambia by Phiri et al.in 2002 and in Nigeria by Gweba et al. 2010, these authors observed prevalences of 20.60% and 14.40% respectively. The prevalence is lower than the 2% reported by Zoli et *al.*[22] in 2003 in their work "Etat régional, épidémiologie et impact de la cysticercose à *Taenia solium* dans les pays occidentaux et Afrique centrale" [Regional status, epidemiology and impact of *Taenia solium* cysticercosis in Western countries and Central Africa]. on the other hand, it is higher than the 0.87% prevalence observed in Benin by Goussanou et *al.*[33] in 2014 cited by Dahourou et *al.*[16] in 2018. However, the difference is very large with the 34% rate observed by Assana et *al.*[9] in 2001 at post-mortem inspection, who worked on the prevalence of cysticercosis in Mayi-Danay (northern Cameroon) and Mayo-Kabbi (south-western Chad). This difference is also very large, with the 20% rate reported by (Phiri et *al.*[66] 2003), observed in post-mortem slaughterhouse inspections in six of Zambia's nine provinces. Our overall prevalence is also higher than the overall prevalences observed in southern Senegal (0.1%) and Gambia (0.2%) by Secka et *al.*[84] in 2010; and in Burkina Faso (0.22%) by Dahourou et al. (2018). All the results obtained at post-mortem examination confirm the presence of cysticercosis in Burkina Faso in general and in the AFO in particular.

This difference could be explained by the Ag-ELISA's sensitivity of 100% (95% CI: 19.79- 100.00) and specificity of 96.4% (95% CI: 90.49- 98.84). [55]In addition, Msawenkosi I Sithole et *al.*[55] reported a higher prevalence (5%) in the Eastern Cape province of South Africa in 2019.In a systematic review in 2015 Kabululu et *al.* [37]in the Mbeya region, Tanzania, the prevalence of *Taenia solium* cysticercosis was 11.5%, according to Ag-ELISA tests. Tassou et *al.* reported an overall prevalence of 7.83% in Benin based on ante-mortem (tongue examination) and post-mortem (health inspection) examinations.[89]Rasamoelina et *al.* provided prevalences of 3.9% using the same method on a study conducted in Madagascar in 2013.[78]These higher prevalences may be explained by the fairly high sensitivity of the ELISA method (92.3%) compared with the conventional method, which detects only a proportion of infected pigs. Variations in prevalence ratios between developed and developing countries are probably due to control efforts such as strict meat inspection regulations and public awareness. Differences in swine cysticercosis prevalence could be explained by agro-climatic conditions, husbandry and climatic conditions, variations in personal and environmental hygiene, correct use of latrines and religion.

In our study, the most infected organ was the heart, with a frequency of 82.0%. The frequency for the tongue was 3.0%. Mopoundza et *al.*[52] in 2019 in Brazaville, in a study of the prevalence of *Taenia solium* cysticercosis in pigs, showed that cysticerci were present in high numbers on the gluteal muscles, followed by the shoulder, masseter and tongue muscles. This difference may be explained by the greater visibility of macroscopic lesions due to the early inflammatory response of the cardiac muscle.

Maeda et *al.*[46] in Tanzania, in a study on the distribution of *T. saginata* cysticerci in cattle organs, also showed that the heart was the most infected organ. These data show that greater care is needed when searching for cysticerci in the heart during post-mortem inspection.

Different data were found in 2010 at the Maroua slaughterhouse in northern Cameroon by Thys, E. [90] who reported a higher frequency in the tongue at 44.17%, while the frequency of cysticercosis in the heart was 26.96%.

The occurrence of porcine cysticercosis in pigs is a major risk factor for *T. solium* taeniasis in humans, particularly in the absence of proper meat inspection practices aimed at treating or condemning infected carcasses and organs before releasing them for human consumption. These treatment and condemnation practices are essential to break the parasite's life cycle. Key factors contributing to disease transmission in Burkina-Faso include free grazing, consumption of raw or undercooked pork, poor personal hygiene practices, lack of consumer awareness of the importance of the disease and its cycle[48].

Although the proportion (1.4%) of cysticercosis-positive pigs was relatively low, the few positive pigs had a high frequency of cysts widely distributed between body and carcass organs. Each positive pig had five cysts. The fact that few animals had high rates of infestation with cysts widely distributed throughout the body has important implications for public health. For example, meat derived from a single animal is consumed collectively by many people in most parts of the country, potentially exposing more people to infection. Indeed, this behavioral practice could explain the high frequency of human taeniasis occurrence in the study area. Our findings of a 1.4% prevalence of porcine cysticercosis on the one hand, and the 9.7% of respondents reporting a previous tapeworm infection on the other, support this hypothesis. More than half the cysts were viable, suggesting that these cysts have the potential to develop into adult worms and cause tapeworm disease when ingested by humans.

IV.3 Socio-demographic characteristics

IV.3.1. Sex and age

In terms of socio-demographics, the population included in our study was 54.7% female. This proportion of women in our study was close to that carried out in 2017 in the DRC by Madinga et *al.* who reported a percentage of women of 55.2% [45].

In addition, different data were reported in 2022 in Madagascar by Rahantamalala et *al.*[75] which showed a higher percentage of men(51.2%) and in 2013 in Tanzania by Mwanjali et *al* (57.4%*)* [56],

According to the RGPH, Ouagadougou has a predominantly female population. The percentage of women in our study can therefore be explained by the higher number of women, but also by the greater ease with which women take part in the surveys.

IV.3.2. Profession and level of education

In terms of level of education, the predominant level was higher education, representing 68.8% of the study population. These data differed from those of studies conducted by Nyangi et al. [63] in 2022 and by Mwanjali et *al*[56] in 2013 in Tanzania, which reported a high level of primary education compared with other levels. These differences in levels between the studies could be explained by the fact that the studies conducted in Tanzania were in rural settings, whereas our study took place in urban settings.

These results, according to our analysis, show that the population has a certain level of understanding that can facilitate awareness-raising on preventive measures for taeniasis. It is therefore important to design specific education programs aimed at informing and protecting the population so that they can understand and appropriate all prevention methods.

With regard to occupation, our study showed a high percentage among housewives (32.2%), followed by pupils and students (31.4%). Different data were reported by Zafindraibe et *al*. [100]in 2017 in Madagascar finding that the majority of the population were students (41.3%), followed by farmers and agriculturists (13.5%).   A study by OA Akinboade[29] on female unemployment in Africa showed that unemployment is higher among women. This may be one explanation for the higher proportion of housewives and shopkeepers.

IV.3.3. Knowledge of tapeworms and eating habits

The proportion (9.7%) of people who reported having had taeniasis in the past is comparable to previous studies reporting 12.5% in Burundi by Minani et *al*.[50] in 2021 and 10% in Vietnam by Ng-Nguyen et *al*. [60]in 2017. On the other hand, the present study showed a lower history of infection compared with these previous studies, including 30% in Indonesia by Wandra et *al.*[96] in 2013, 28.48% in Thailand by kusolsuk et *al.* in 2021[42]. Our study indicates that human taeniasis is a major public health problem that could be attributed to the lack of routine meat inspection policy by trained inspectors and a high rate of raw or undercooked meat consumption in the population (51.5%). Indeed, those who consumed undercooked meat were 25 times more likely to have reported a history of previous tapeworm infection than those who did not. Our results also suggest that cooking meat before consumption is a simple, affordable and effective way to protect against infection. However, changing meat consumption practices requires an awareness campaign to educate the public about the risk associated with eating raw meat in the study area and in the country in general. Although half of the respondents are aware of the need to prevent taeniasis through public education and meat inspection services, better access to basic hygiene and sanitation facilities is still needed.

As for their knowledge of *T. solium*, a wide range of information was found. The majority of respondents had already heard of the disease (84.20%). This may be due to the fact that more than half the respondents had a higher level of education. Similar data were reported by Mwindunda et *al.*[57] in 2015 in Brazzaville.

However, the routes of transmission and the agent responsible for taeniasis are unknown to most people, Dahourou et *al.*[16] reported similar data in 2018 in the Boucle du Mouhoun region. In the study by Ngowi et *al.*[61]in Burkina Faso, only 5.3% of people were aware that tapeworm infestation is associated with the consumption of raw infected pork. Chacha et *al.*[15]in Tanzania and Ngowi et *al.*[61] in Burkina Faso found respectively that 33.7% and 6.2% of the population were aware that porcine cysticercosis is linked to the consumption of human faeces by pigs. This lack of knowledge of cysticercosis transmission among the population in our study area is dangerous, as a good understanding of *T. solium* transmission to the population and to pigs makes it possible to avoid human behaviors that increase the risk of transmission to both humans and pigs.

Indeed, a lack of knowledge among the population about the epidemiology of porcine and human cysticercosis leads to behaviors that facilitate the transmission and maintenance of *T. solium* infections[87]. This situation justifies the fact that 23.8% of the population is unaware that eating infected raw meat can make them ill. Thus, it appears that the population of the area is aware of the disease, but the epidemiology remains unknown. This situation was also observed by Shey-Njila et *al.*[85]in Cameroon. Contrary to our study, which revealed a percentage of 45% of consumers with knowledge of the causal agent of taeniasis, Ngowi et *al.*[61] and Garcia et al.[26] reported that 28.6% of the population was aware of the relationship between tapeworm disease in humans and cysticercosis. Lack of awareness of the tapeworm/cysticercosis pair makes it difficult to control in endemic areas. Moreover, Lazare et *al.*[43] showed that educating the population was associated with a reduction in the incidence of porcine cysticercosis. This study shows that people are aware of the existence of cysticercosis, but are unaware of its epidemiology and the potential risk of human infestation by infected pigs, but also by humans carrying the adult worm. It is therefore very important to raise awareness among local populations of the transmission of *T. solium* to pigs and humans.

Some of those surveyed claimed to have experienced discomfort after eating pork. These were characterized by headaches, convulsions, vomiting, diarrhea, stomach ache, often followed by bloating and buzzing in the stomach. Similar data have been reported by Wu[98] in a study of the various hazards associated with pork consumption.

We have estimated the number of people likely to be infected with tapeworms through the consumption of uninspected meat or carcasses contaminated with cysticerci. In theory, a single larva is capable of infecting a human. The data from our study revealed dietary practices and habits highly at risk of contamination in the study population. Considering that a large proportion of the study population (71%) often consumed meat that had not been inspected by veterinary services, and that 51.5% of the study population stated that they often consumed undercooked or raw meat.

It appears that the number of people likely to be infected with taeniasis is very high (on average 40 to 60% of the study population).

CONCLUSION

CONCLUSION

Swine cysticercosis is a common parasitic disease in many parts of the world, which can have serious consequences for human health. Risk factors for *Taenia solium* taeniasis in pork consumers include the consumption of undercooked or raw pork, as well as inadequate sanitary conditions during the rearing, handling and preparation of pork.

To prevent swine cysticercosis and *Taenia solium* tapeworm among pork consumers, it is essential to improve public health and food safety policies, as well as pork farming and preparation practices, in particular by raising public awareness of the risks associated with eating raw or undercooked meat.

In addition, further research is needed to assess the effectiveness of different public health interventions, particularly in those parts of the world where swine cysticercosis and *Taenia solium* tapeworm are most prevalent. Ultimately, it is imperative that governments and regulators work together to ensure public health and safety, and to mitigate the risks associated with pork consumption.

The world is currently facing an upsurge in infectious and non-infectious diseases, capable of affecting the global health system. According to statistics, around 75% of new diseases affecting humans in the last ten (10) years are due to pathogens originating from animals or animal products.

The painful episodes of the Ebola virus disease epidemic that raged in West Africa between 2014 and 2016 produced a death toll of over 25,000 cases, including more than 11,000 deaths. This epidemic demonstrated the fragility of our systems for monitoring, preventing and controlling health risks of all origins. In addition, the lacklustre management of this epidemic demonstrated the need to reconsider the vision of human health and to apprehend it in the complexity of its interactions with animal and environmental health, with the implementation of the One Health approach. Nevertheless, the experience we have gained has enabled us to deal more rapidly with the Ebola Virus infection of 2021 in the Republic of Guinea.

Thus, in 2014, over 60 countries, international organizations and non-governmental organizations launched the Global Health Security Action Program (or GHSA in English), whose aim is to help countries strengthen their capacities to help protect the world from epidemic threats and achieve global health security as a priority. The program is now the main tool for implementing the directives of the International Health Regulations (IHR 2005) in a One Health approach.

Burkina Faso signed up to the Global Health Security Agenda in 2016

RECOMMENDATIONS

Suggestion s

In order to reduce the morbidity of *T. solium* taeniasis and promote the health of the population, and in view of the many risks present, we suggest that appropriate personal and collective hygiene measures be reinforced, in particular:

- Health education on hygiene and environmental sanitation. Inform and sensitize breeders on intensive breeding to avoid repeated wandering and infestation of animals.
- Educating the public about the dangers of clandestine slaughter
- Reinforcing systematic deworming
- Improved screening, treatment and prevention services
- A much more rigorous approach to carcass inspection

In view of the above, we recommend :

- The ministry in charge, to promote concrete actions in terms of environmental health and sanitation;
- To the Ministry of Public Health, to organize and intensify mass health education to effectively combat fecal peril, clandestine slaughter and fraud;
- It's up to people to be more demanding about where their meat comes from and to cook it thoroughly before eating;
- Health professionals should consider similar studies in other parts of the country to obtain more precise data on the various aspects of these parasitic diseases.

REFERENCES

REFERENCES

1. **Abunna F, Tilahun G, Megersa B, Regassa A, Kumsa B**. Bovine cysticercosis in cattle slaughtered at Awassa municipal abattoir, Ethiopia: Zoonoses Public Health. 2008;55(2):82-8.

2. **Adalid-Peralta L, Rosas G, Arce-Sillas A, Bobes RJ, Cárdenas G, Hernández M, *et al*.** Effect of Transforming Growth Factor-β upon Taenia solium and Taenia crassiceps Cysticerci. Sci Rep. 27 Sep 2017 ;7(1) :12345.

3. **Akinboade OA**. Women, poverty and informal trade in Eastern and Southern Africa. International Social Science Journal. 2005 ;184(2) :277-300.

4. **Andriantsimahavandy A, Lesbordes JL, Rasoaharimalala B, Peghini M, Rabarijaona L, Roux J,*et al*.** Neurocysticercosis: a major aetiological factor of late-onset epilepsy in Madagascar. Trop Med Int Health. August 1997;2(8):741-6.

5. **Anjanirina R, Porphyre V, Rabenindrina N, Julien R, Andriamanivo H, Jambou R**. Cysticercosis, a neglected disease. In 2016. p. 309-45.

6. **Arana Y, Verastegui M, Tuero I, Grandjean L, Garcia HH, Gilman RH**. Characterization of the carbohydrate components of Taenia solium oncosphere proteins and their role in the antigenicity. Parasitol Res. Oct 2013;112(10):3569-78.

7. **Arriola CS, Gonzalez AE, Gomez-Puerta LA, Lopez-Urbina MT, Garcia HH, Gilman RH**. New insights into cysticercosis transmission. PLoS Negl Trop Dis. Oct 2014;8(10):e3247.

8. **van As AD, Joubert J**. Neurocysticercosis in 578 black epileptic patients. S Afr Med J. 5 Oct 1991;80(7):327-8.

9. **Assana E, Amadou F, Thys E, Lightowlers MW, Zoli AP, Dorny P, *et al*.** Pig-farming systems and porcine cysticercosis in the north of Cameroon. J Helminthol. Dec 2010;84(4):441-6.

10. **Bizhani n, Bashemi hafshejani s, Mohammadi n, Mezaei m, Rokni mb**. Human Cysticercosis in Asia: A Systematic Review and Meta-Analysis. Iran J Public Health. oct 2020;49(10):1839-47.

11. **Bouilliant-Linet E, Brugières P, Coubes P, Gaston A, Laporte P, Marsault C**. [Cerebral cysticercosis. Diagnostic value of x-ray computed tomography. Apropos of 117 cases]. J Radiol. 1988;69(6-7):405-12.

12. **Burneo JG, Plener I, Garcia HH**. Neurocysticercosis in a patient in Canada. CMAJ. March 17, 2009;180(6):639-42.

13. **Bustos JA, Rodriguez S, Jimenez JA, Moyano LM, Castillo Y, Ayvar V, *et al*. Cysticercosis Working Group in Peru**. Detection of Taenia solium taeniasis coproantigen is an early indicator of treatment failure for taeniasis. Clin Vaccine Immunol. Apr 2012 ;19(4):570-3.

14. **Canada A of Public Health**. Fiche Technique Santé-Sécurité : Agents Pathogènes - Taenia solium mai 2023,15(9):679-6.

15. **Chacha M, Yohana C, Nkwengulila G**. Indigenous Knowledge, Practices, Beliefs and Social Impacts of Porcine Cysticercosis and Epilepsy in Iringa Rural. Health. 23 Dec 2014;6(21):2894-903.

16. **Dahourou LD, Gbati OB, Millogo A, Dicko A, Roamba CR, Pangui LJ**. Analysis of the Knowledge, Attitudes and Practices of Populations in

Four Villages of the *Boucle du Mouhoun* Region (Burkina Faso) Regarding *Taenia solium* Life Cycle. Health. 18 Jan 2018;10(01):95.

17. **Deckers N, Dorny P**. Immunodiagnosis of Taenia solium taeniosis/cysticercosis. Trends Parasitol. March 2010;26(3):137-44.

18. **DeGiorgio C, Pietsch-Escueta S, Tsang V, Corral-Leyva G, Ng L, Medina MT, Astudillo S, *et al***. Sero-prevalence of Taenia solium cysticercosis and Taenia solium taeniasis in California, USA. Acta Neurol Scand. Feb 2005;111(2):84-8.

19. **Derakhshani A, Mousavi SM, Rezaei M, Afgar A, Keyhani AR, Mohammadi MA, *et al***. Natural history of Echinococcus granulosus microcyst development in long term in vitro culture and molecular and morphological changes induced by insulin and BMP-4. Front Vet Sci. 2022; 9:1068602.

20. **Engels D, Urbani C, Belotto A, Meslin F, Savioli L**. The control of human (neuro)cysticercosis: which way forward? Acta Trop. June 2003;87(1):177-82.

21. **Eshitera EE, Githigia SM, Kitala P, Thomas LF, Fèvre EM, Harrison LJS, *et al***. Prevalence of porcine cysticercosis and associated risk factors in Homa Bay District, Kenya. BMC Vet Res. Dec 5, 2012; 8:234.

22. **Ev K, Ec K, Ha N, Si K, Je M, Fp L, *et al***. Prevalence of porcine cysticercosis and associated risk factors in smallholder pig production systems in Mbeya region, southern highlands of Tanzania. Veterinary parasitology. June 12, 2013;198(3-4):45.

23. **Flisser A, Rodríguez-Canul R, Willingham AL**. Control of the taeniosis/cysticercosis complex: future developments. Vet Parasitol. 31 Jul 2006;139(4):283-92.

24. **Flisser A, Sarti E, Lightowlers M, Schantz P**. Neurocysticercosis: regional status, epidemiology, impact and control measures in the Americas. Acta Trop. June 2003;87(1):43-51.

25. **Gajadhar AA, Scandrett WB, Forbes LB**. Overview of food- and water-borne zoonotic parasites at the farm level. Rev Sci Tech. August 2006;25(2):595-606.

26. **García HH, González AE, Del Brutto OH, Tsang VCW, Llanos-Zavalaga F, Gonzalvez G, *et al***. Strategies for the elimination of taeniasis/cysticercosis. J Neurol Sci. 15 Nov 2007;262(1-2):153-7.

27. **García HH, Gonzalez AE, Evans CAW, Gilman RH, Cysticercosis Working Group in Peru**. Taenia solium cysticercosis. Lancet. August 16, 2003;362(9383):547-56.

28. **Garcia HH, O'Neal SE, Noh J, Handali S, Cysticercosis Working Group in Peru**. Laboratory Diagnosis of Neurocysticercosis (Taenia solium). J Clin Microbiol. Sept 2018;56(9):e00424-18.

29. **Garcia-Noval J, Allan JC, Fletes C, Moreno E, DeMata F, Torres-Alvarez R, *et al***. Epidemiology of Taenia solium taeniasis and cysticercosis in two rural Guatemalan communities. Am J Trop Med Hyg. Sept 1996;55(3):282-9.

30. **Gonzales I, Rivera JT, Garcia HH, Cysticercosis Working Group in Peru**. Pathogenesis of Taenia solium taeniasis and cysticercosis. Parasite Immunol. March 2016;38(3):136-46.

31. **Gonzalez AE, Cama V, Gilman RH, Tsang VC, Pilcher JB, Chavera A, *et al***. Prevalence and comparison of serologic assays, necropsy, and

tongue examination for the diagnosis of porcine cysticercosis in Peru. Am J Trop Med Hyg. August 1990;43(2):194-9.

32. **Gonzalez AE, Lopez-Urbina T, Tsang B, Gavidia C, Garcia HH, Silva ME,** *et al*. Transmission dynamics of Taenia solium and potential for pig-to-pig transmission. Parasitol Int. 2006;55 Suppl: S131-135.

33. **Goussanou JSE, Korsak N, Saegerman C, Youssao AKI, Azagoun E, Farougou S,** *et al*. Assessment of Routine Inspection Method for Diagnosis of Porcine Cysticercosis in South East Benin by Using Meat Inspection Records and Ag-ELISA Test. International Journal of Animal and Veterinary Advances. apr 2014;6(2):80-6.

34. **Huerta M, Avila R, Jiménez HI, Díaz R, Díaz J, Díaz Huerta ME,** *et al*. Parasite contamination of soil in households of a Mexican rural community endemic for neurocysticercosis. Trans R Soc Trop Med Hyg. Apr 2008;102(4):374-9.

35. **Ito A, Wandra T, Yamasaki H, Nakao M, Sako Y, Nakaya K,** *et al*. Cysticercosis/taeniasis in Asia and the Pacific. Vector Borne Zoonotic Dis. 2004;4(2):95-107.

36. **Kabululu ML, Johansen MV, Mlangwa JED, Mkupasi EM, Braae UC, Trevisan C,** *et al*. Performance of Ag-ELISA in the diagnosis of Taenia solium cysticercosis in naturally infected pigs in Tanzania. Parasit Vectors. 27 Oct 2020;13(1):534.

37. **Kabululu ML, Ngowi HA, Kimera SI, Lekule FP, Kimbi EC, Johansen MV.** Risk factors for prevalence of pig parasitoses in Mbeya Region, Tanzania. Vet Parasitol. 15 Sep 2015;212(3-4):460-4.

38. **Karki G**. Taenia solium; morphology, life cycle, pathogenesis, clinical infection, lab diagnosis, treatment, prevention and epidemiology. Online Biology Notes. May 2023,667(88). taenia-solium-morphology-life-cycle-pathogenesis-clinical-infection-lab-diagnosis-treatment-prevention-and-epidemiology

39. **Karki G**. Taenia solium; morphology, life cycle, pathogenesis, clinical infection, lab diagnosis, treatment, prevention and epidemiology [Internet]. Online Biology Notes. Apr 2023,55(22):67-88

40. **Krecek RC**. Third meeting of the Cysticercosis Working Group in Eastern and Southern Africa takes place in Maputo. J S Afr Vet Assoc. March 2005;76(1):2-3.

41. **Krecek RC, Mohammed H, Michael LM, Schantz PM, Ntanjana L, Morey L, *et al*.** Risk Factors of Porcine Cysticercosis in the Eastern Cape Province, South Africa. PLoS One. May 24, 2012;7(5): e37718.

42. **Kusolsuk T, Chaisiri K, Poodeepiyasawad A, Sa-Nguankiat S, Homsuwan N, Yanagida T, *et al*.** Risk factors and prevalence of taeniasis among the Karen people of Tha Song Yang District, Tak Province, Thailand. Parasite. 28 :53.

43. **Lazare V**. la taeniose humaine due to taenia solium dans deux groupements de la menoua (ouest-cameroun).

44. **Lightowlers MW, Colebrook AL, Gauci CG, Gauci SM, Kyngdon CT, *et al*.** Vaccination against cestode parasites: anti-helminth vaccines that work and why. Vet Parasitol. July 25, 2003;115(2):83-123.

45. **Madinga J, Polman K, Kanobana K, van Lieshout L, Brienen E, Praet N, *et al*.** Epidemiology of polyparasitism with Taenia solium, schistosomes and soil-transmitted helminths in the co-endemic village of Malanga, Democratic Republic of Congo. Acta Tropica. 1 Jul 2017; 171:186-93.

46. **Maeda GE, Kyvsgaard NChr, Nansen P, Bøgh HO.** Distribution of Taenia saginata cysts by muscle group in naturally infected cattle in Tanzania. Preventive Veterinary Medicine. 1 Sep 1996;28(2):81-9.

47. **Mafojane NA, Appleton CC, Krecek RC, Michael LM, Willingham AL.** The current status of neurocysticercosis in Eastern and Southern Africa. Acta Trop. June 2003;87(1):25-33.

48. **Megersa B, Tesfaye E, Regassa A, Abebe R, Abunna F.** Bovine cysticercosis in Cattle Slaughtered at Jimma Municipal Abattoir, South western Ethiopia: Prevalence, Cyst viability and Its Socio-economic importance. Vet World. 2010;2(2):257.

49. **Migliani R, Rasolomaharo M, Rajaonarison P, Ravaoalimalala VE, Rabarijaona L, Andriantsimahavandy A.** [Cysticercosis in the port of Mahajanga: more frequent than we thought!]. Arch Inst Pasteur Madagascar. 2000;66(1-2):39-42.

50. **Minani S.** Prevalence and risk assessment of porcine cysticercosis in Ngozi province, Burundi. 2021;

51. **Moore AC, Lutwick LI, Schantz PM, Pilcher JB, Wilson M, Hightower AW, *et al*.** Seroprevalence of cysticercosis in an Orthodox Jewish community. Am J Trop Med Hyg. Nov 1995;53(5):439-42.

52. **Mopoundza P, Missoko RM, Angandza GS, Mbou AS, Akouango P.** Prevalence of Taenia solium (Cysticercus cellulosae) porcine cysticercosis in pigs in the slaughtering area of Kinsoundi, Brazzaville. International Journal of Biological and Chemical Sciences. Sep 9, 2019;13(3):1396-410.

53. **Morales J, Martínez JJ, Rosetti M, Fleury A, Maza V, Hernandez M,** *et al.* Spatial Distribution of Taenia solium Porcine Cysticercosis within a Rural Area of Mexico. PLoS Negl Trop Dis. 3 sept 2008 ;2(9) : e284.

54. **Murrell D.** Zoonotic foodborne parasites and their surveillance. Scientific and Technical Review (International Office of Epizootics). August 1, 2013; 32:559-69.

55. **Mwabonimana M-F, King'ori AM, Inyagwa CM, Shakala EK, Bebe BO.** PREVALENCE OF PORCINE CYSTICERCOSIS AMONG SCAVENGING PIGS IN WESTERN KENYA. Afr J Infect Dis. 2020;14(2):30-5.

56. **Mwanjali G, Kihamia C, Kakoko DVC, Lekule F, Ngowi H, Johansen MV,** *et al.* Prevalence and Risk Factors Associated with Human Taenia Solium Infections in Mbozi District, Mbeya Region, Tanzania. PLOS Neglected Tropical Diseases. March 14, 2013;7(3): e2102.

57. **Mwidunda SA, Carabin H, Matuja WBM, Winkler AS, Ngowi HA.** A School Based Cluster Randomised Health Education Intervention Trial for Improving Knowledge and Attitudes Related to Taenia solium Cysticercosis and Taeniasis in Mbulu District, Northern Tanzania. PLOS ONE. Feb 26, 2015;10(2): e0118541.

58. **Naidoo DV, Pammenter MD, Moosa A, van Dellen JR, Cosnett JE.** Seventy black epileptics. Cysticercosis, computed tomography and electro-encephalography. S Afr Med J. Dec 19, 1987;72(12):837-8.

59. **Ndri KT-B, Razafiarimanga ZN, Randriamparany T, Nowakowsky M, Djaman JA, Jambou R.** Prevalence of porcine cysticercosis in three slaughterhouses in Antananarivo, Madagascar: comparison of carcass inspection versus serological testing.

60. **Ng-Nguyen D, Stevenson MA, Traub RJ**. A systematic review of taeniasis, cysticercosis and trichinellosis in Vietnam. Parasit Vectors. 2017 March 21;10(1):150.

61. **Ngowi H, Ozbolt I, Millogo A, Dermauw V, Somé T, Spicer P, *et al***. Development of a health education intervention strategy using an implementation research method to control taeniasis and cysticercosis in Burkina Faso. Infect Dis Poverty. 1 June 2017;6(1):95.

62. **Nguekam JP, Zoli AP, Zogo PO, Kamga ACT, Speybroeck N, Dorny P, *et al***. A seroepidemiological study of human cysticercosis in West Cameroon. Tropical Medicine & International Health. 2003;8(2):144-9.

63. **Nyangi C, Stelzle D, Mkupasi EM, Ngowi HA, Churi AJ, Schmidt V, *et al***. Knowledge, attitudes and practices related to Taenia solium cysticercosis and taeniasis in Tanzania. BMC Infectious Diseases. June 13, 2022;22(1):534.

64. **Pawlowski Z, Allan J, Sarti E**. Control of Taenia solium taeniasis/cysticercosis: from research towards implementation. Int J Parasitol. Oct 2005;35(11-12):1221-32.

65. **Pawłowski ZS**. Efficacy of low doses of praziquantel in taeniasis. Acta Trop. Dec 1990;48(2):83-8.

66. **Phiri IK, Ngowi H, Afonso S, Matenga E, Boa M, Mukaratirwa S, *et al***. The emergence of Taenia solium cysticercosis in Eastern and Southern Africa as a serious agricultural problem and public health risk. Acta Trop. June 2003;87(1):13-23.

67. **Pondja A, Neves L, Mlangwa J, Afonso S, Fafetine J, Willingham AL, *et al***. Prevalence and risk factors of porcine cysticercosis in Angónia District, Mozambique. PLoS Negl Trop Dis. Feb 2, 2010;4(2): e594.

68. **Porphyre V, Rasamoelina-Andriamanivo H, Rakotoarimanana A, Rasamoelina O, Bernard C, Jambou R,** *et al.* Spatio-temporal prevalence of porcine cysticercosis in Madagascar based on meat inspection. Parasit Vectors. 25 Jul 2015; 8:391.

69. **Pouedet MSR, Zoli AP, Nguekam null, Vondou L, Assana E, Speybroeck N, Berkvens D,** *et al.* Epidemiological survey of swine cysticercosis in two rural communities of West-Cameroon. Vet Parasitol. May 30, 2002;106(1):45-54.

70. **Pouedet MSR, Zoli AP, Nguekam null, Vondou L, Assana E, Speybroeck N,** *et al.* Epidemiological survey of swine cysticercosis in two rural communities of West-Cameroon. Vet Parasitol. May 30, 2002;106(1):45-54.

71. **Prasad KN, Prasad A, Verma A, Singh AK.** Human cysticercosis and Indian scenario: a review. J Biosci. Nov 2008;33(4):571-82.

72. **Preiser W.** Hartmut Krauss, Albert Weber, Max Appel, Burkhard Enders, Henry D. Isenberg, Hans Gerd Schiefer, Werner Slenczka, Alexander von Graevenitz, and Horst Zahner. Zoonoses: infectious diseases transmissible from animals to humans, 3rd edition. Med Microbiol Immunol. 2005 ;194(4) :219-20.

73. **Quet F, Guerchet M, Pion SDS, Ngoungou EB, Nicoletti A, Preux P-M.** Meta-analysis of the association between cysticercosis and epilepsy in Africa. Epilepsia. May 2010;51(5):830-7.

74. **Rahantamalala A, Porphyre V, Rabenindrina N, Razafimahefa J, Rasamoelina-Andriamanivo H, Jambou R.** La cysticercose une maladie négligée Cysticercosis a neglected disease.

75. **Rahantamalala A, Rakotoarison RL, Rakotomalala E, Rakotondrazaka M, Kiernan J, Castle PM,** *et al.* Prevalence and factors associated with human Taenia solium taeniosis and cysticercosis in twelve remote villages of Ranomafana rainforest, Madagascar. PLoS Negl Trop Dis. 11 Apr 2022;16(4):e0010265.

76. **Raïssa F, Jacques N.** Persistence of Tenia solium amongst others human Gastro-intestinal parasites in Bamboutos locality (West region-Cameroon). JABs. 27 Dec 2019; 144:14813-21.

77. **Rasamoelina-Andriamanivo H, Porphyre V, Jambou R.** Control of cysticercosis in Madagascar: beware of the pitfalls. Trends Parasitol. nov 2013 ;29(11) :538-47.

78. **Rasamoelina-Andriamanivo H, Rasamoelina EO, Porphyre V.** Study of the importance of cysticercosis in Madagascar by monitoring slaughterhouses [Internet]. Journées scientifiques qualiREG. 3rd edition. QualiREG. QualiREG Food Symposium. Food quality in the Indian Ocean.2013 June 8, 2023.

79. **Román G, Sotelo J, Del Brutto O, Flisser A, Dumas M, Wadia N,***et al.* A proposal to declare neurocysticercosis an international reportable disease. Bull World Health Organ. 2000;78(3):399-406.

80. **Saini PK, Webert DW, McCASKEY PC.** Food Safety and Regulatory Aspects of Cattle and Swine Cysticercosis. J Food Prot. Apr 1997;60(4):447-53.

81. **Sarti E, Schantz PM, Plancarte A, Wilson M, Gutierrez OI, Aguilera J,** *et al.* Epidemiological investigation of Taenia solium taeniasis and cysticercosis in a rural village of Michoacan state, Mexico. Trans R Soc Trop Med Hyg. 1994;88(1):49-52.

82. **Schantz PM, Moore AC, Muñoz JL, Hartman BJ, Schaefer JA, Aron AM, *et al*.** Neurocysticercosis in an Orthodox Jewish community in New York City. N Engl J Med. 3 Sep 1992;327(10):692-5.

83. **Sciutto E, Chavarria A, Fragoso G, Fleury A, Larralde C**. The immune response in Taenia solium cysticercosis: protection and injury. Parasite Immunol. Dec 2007;29(12):621-36.

84. **Secka A, Marcotty T, De Deken R, Van Marck E, Geerts S**. Porcine cysticercosis and risk factors in the gambia and senegal. J Parasitol Res. 2010; 2010:823892.

85. **Shey-Njila O, Zoli PA, Awah-Ndukum J, Nguekam null, Assana E, Byambas P, *et al*.** Porcine cysticercosis in village pigs of North-West Cameroon. J Helminthol. Dec 2003;77(4):351-4.

86. **Sinha S, Sharma BS**. Neurocysticercosis: a review of current status and management. J Clin Neurosci. Jul 2009;16(7):867-76.

87. **Sorvillo F, Wilkins P, Shafir S, Eberhard M**. Public health implications of cysticercosis acquired in the United States. Emerg Infect Dis. Jan 2011;17(1):1-6.

88. **Sorvillo FJ, DeGiorgio C, Waterman SH**. Deaths from Cysticercosis, United States. Emerg Infect Dis. Feb 2007;13(2):230-5.

89. **Tassou AW, Attindehou S, Gbati OB, Montchowui HE, Salifou S**. Prevalence of porcine cysticercosis in informal slaughtering areas in Benin. Sciences and Technologies for Substainable Agriculture. June 27, 2022 ;2(1) :30-5.

90. **Thys E**. Contribution à l'étude de la cysticercose bovine à l'abattoir de Maroua. TROPICULTURA. 1(1):13-2o.

91. **Tolosa T, Tigre W, Teka G, Dorny P**. Prevalence of bovine cysticercosis and hydatidosis in Jimma municipal abattoir, South West Ethiopia. Onderstepoort J Vet Res. Sept 2009;76(3):323-6.

92. **Tsegaye D, Gutema FD, Terefe Y**. Zoonotic diseases risk perceptions and protective behaviors of consumers associated with consumption of meat and milk in and around Bishoftu, Ethiopia. Heliyon. August 2022;8(8): e10351.

93. **Tsotetsi-Khambule AM, Njiro S, Katsande TC, Harrison LJS**. Risk factors associated with taeniosis-cysticercosis in rural farming communities in Gauteng Province, South Africa. Trop Anim Health Prod. Dec 2018;50(8):1951-5.

94. **Vondou L, Zoli AP, Nguekam null, Pouedet S, Assana E, Kamga Tokam AC, Dorny P, *et al***. [Taenia solium taeniasis/cysticercosis in the Menoua division (West Cameroon)]. Parasite. Sept 2002;9(3):271-4.

95. **Vondou L, Zoli AP, Pouedet S, Assana E, Tokam ACK, Dorny P, *et al***. Taenia solium taeniosis/cysticercosis in Menoua (West Cameroon). Parasite. 1 Sep 2002;9(3):271-4.

96. **Wandra T, Ito A, Swastika K, Dharmawan NS, Sako Y, Okamoto M**. Taeniases and cysticercosis in Indonesia: past and present situations. Parasitology. nov 2013;140(13):1608-16.

97. **Willingham AL, Harrison LJ, Fèvre EM, Parkhouse ME**. Inaugural Meeting of the Cysticercosis Working Group in Europe1. Emerg Infect Dis. Dec 2008;14(12):e2.

98. **Wu W, Qian X, Huang Y, Hong Q**. A review of the control of clonorchiasis sinensis and Taenia solium taeniasis/cysticercosis in China. Parasitol Res. Nov 2012;111(5):1879-84.

99. **Yanagida T, Yuzawa I, Joshi DD, Sako Y, Nakao M, Nakaya K, *et al*.** Neurocysticercosis: assessing where the infection was acquired from. J Travel Med. 2010 ;17(3):206-8.

100. **Zafindraibe NJ, Ralalarinivo J, Rakotoniaina AI, Maeder MN, Andrianarivelo MR, Contamin B, *et al*.** Seroprevalence of cysticercosis and associated risk factors in a group of patients seen at the Centre Hospitalier Régional de Référence d'Antsirabe, Madagascar. Pan Afr Med J. Nov 23, 2017; 28:260.

101. **Zammarchi L, Bonati M, Strohmeyer M, Albonico M, Requena-Méndez A, Bisoffi Z, *et al*.** Screening, diagnosis and management of human cysticercosis and Taenia solium taeniasis: technical recommendations by the COHEMI project study group. Trop Med Int Health. Jul 2017;22(7):881-94.

102. **Zoli A, Shey-Njila O, Assana E, Nguekam J-P, Dorny P, Brandt J, Geerts S**. Regional status, epidemiology and impact of Taenia solium cysticercosis in Western and Central Africa. Acta Trop. June 2003;87(1):35-42.

103. WER8613_113-120.pdf [Internet]. [cited June 9, 2023]. Available from: https://apps.who.int/iris/bitstream/handle/10665/241731/WER8613_113-120.PDF

104. Bourée P, Dahane N, Resende P, Bisaro F, Ensaf A. Cestodes and their laboratory diagnosis. Revue Francophone des Laboratoires. March 2012;2012(440):67-73.

105.   Brandt JR, Geerts S, De Deken R, Kumar V, Ceulemans F, Brijs L, Falla N. A monoclonal antibody-based ELISA for the detection of circulating excretory-secretory antigens in Taenia saginata cysticercosis. Int J Parasitol. July 1992;22(4):471-7.

106..   Fahmy HA, Khalifa NO, EL-Madawy RS, Afify JSA, Aly NSM, Kandil OM. Prevalence of Bovine Cysticercosis and Taenia saginata in Man. 2015;

APPENDICES

APPENDICES

<u>**Teniasis questionnaire**</u>

Gender

Male ☐ Female☐

Age

- ☐ 15-25 years
- ☐ 26-35 years
- ☐ 36-45years
- ☐ 46-55 years old
- ☐ Over 55

Study level

....

....

Profession

- ☐ Student
- ☐ Student
- ☐ Civil servant
- ☐ Retailer
- ☐ Housekeeper
- ☐ Other :

Area of residence

....

....

Have you ever heard of tapeworm or any other parasite-related illness associated with eating pork?

- ☐ YES
- ☐ NO

Do you know the causes of tapeworm?

- ☐ YES
- ☐ NO

Did you know that *Taenia solium* is the agent responsible for swine cysticercosis?

☐ YES
☐ NO

Do you know the symptoms of *Taenia solium* tapeworm in humans?

☐ YES
☐ NO

Do you know the human health risks associated with eating undercooked or raw pork?

☐ YES
☐ NO

Have you ever experienced symptoms such as headaches, abdominal pain or digestive problems after eating pork?

☐ YES
☐ NO

Have you ever been diagnosed with *Taenia solium* tapeworm?

☐ YES
☐ NO

Do you know how to prevent tapeworm?

☐ YES
☐ NO

Do you have any suggestions for improving awareness of tapeworm prevention in your community?

....

Do you have any other questions or comments about taeniasis that you'd like to share?

....

How often do you eat pork?

....

Can you estimate the average cost of pork you consume per week?

- ☐ Less than 500 CFA francs
- ☐ 500 to 2000 CFA francs
- ☐ 2000 to 5000 CFA francs
- ☐ More than 5,000 CFA francs

Where do you buy your meat?

- ☐ At the market
- ☐ In charcuterie
- ☐ Breeders
- ☐ Itinerant butchers
- ☐ At the local butcher's
- ☐ Anywhere

Do you require meat to be inspected by veterinary services before you buy it?

- ☐ YES
- ☐ NO

Do you eat grilled or smoked meat from the tracks? If so, do you usually reheat it before consumption?

....

How do you cook your meat?

- ☐ Grill/Barbecue
- ☐ Oil/oven cooking
- ☐ Water cooking (soup)
- ☐ Frying
- ☐ Other

Do you eat imported meat?

Have you ever eaten undercooked or raw meat?

- ☐ YES
- ☐ NO

Collection sheet

Pork	Date of slaughter	Type of breeding	Results of muscle tissue inspection	Infected organs
1				
2				
3				
4				
5				
6				
7				
8				
9				
10				
11				
12				
13				
14				
15				

ICONOGRAPHY

ICONOGRAPHY

- Infected heart

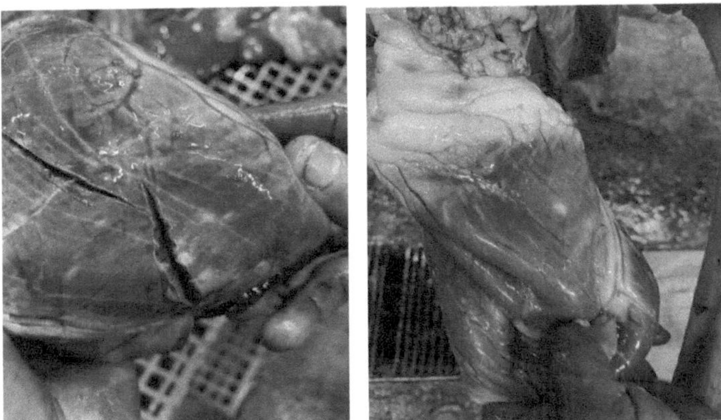

- Slaughter line

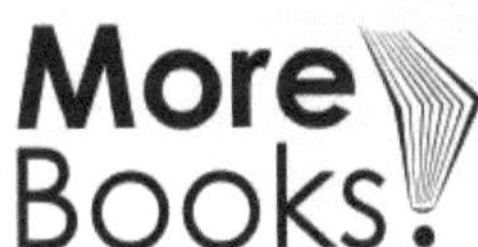

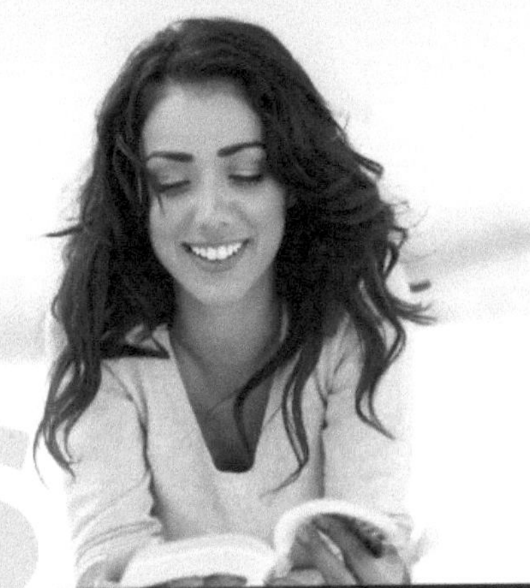

I want morebooks!

Buy your books fast and straightforward online - at one of world's fastest growing online book stores! Environmentally sound due to Print-on-Demand technologies.

Buy your books online at
www.morebooks.shop

Kaufen Sie Ihre Bücher schnell und unkompliziert online – auf einer der am schnellsten wachsenden Buchhandelsplattformen weltweit! Dank Print-On-Demand umwelt- und ressourcenschonend produziert.

Bücher schneller online kaufen
www.morebooks.shop

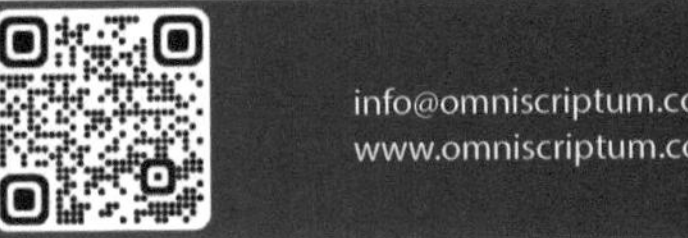

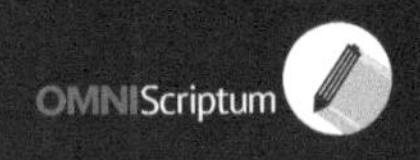

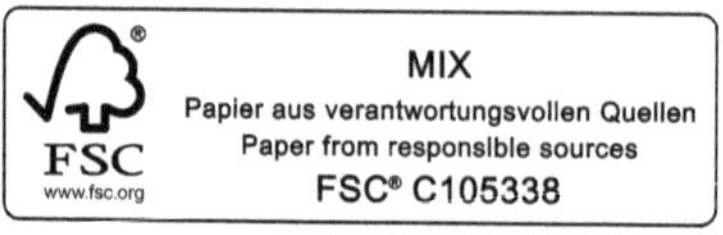

Printed by Books on Demand GmbH, Norderstedt / Germany